Dr Mark Port[

RadioTimes

Complete Lifeplan

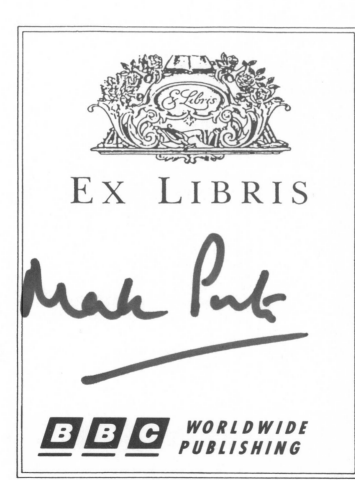

EX LIBRIS

BBC *WORLDWIDE PUBLISHING*

Dr Mark Porter's

RadioTimes

Complete Lifeplan

....

Mark Porter
with Helen Reilly

NETWORK BOOKS

ABOUT THE AUTHORS

On qualifying as a doctor, **Mark Porter** spent five years working in hospital specialist departments before entering general practice and still runs a surgery two days a week. He was appointed assistant medical editor to *General Practitioner* in 1991 and joined BBC's *Good Morning...with Anne and Nick* the following year where he had a twice-weekly slot as its resident doctor until 1996. He is a medical columnist for *Radio Times* and the *Sunday Mirror*, and is the resident doctor on Classic FM's *Newsnight*. Mark and his wife, Ros, live in Gloucestershire with their two young daughters, Charlotte and Sarah.

A graduate of Natural Sciences from Cambridge University, **Helen Reilly** worked as a science news writer on *General Practitioner* until 1993 when she became medical correspondent of the *Sunday Mirror*. Helen lives in London with her partner, Anthony Bullman.

Network Books is an imprint of BBC Books,
a division of BBC Worldwide Publishing,
Woodlands, 80 Wood Lane,
London W12 OTT

First published in 1996
ISBN 0 563 37174 9

Illustrations by Sarah Williams
Ideal weight chart on page 44 reproduced by the kind permission
of the Health Education Authority
Set in Perpetua and Helvetica Neue
Printed by Martins the Printers Ltd, Berwick-upon-Tweed
Bound by Hunter & Foulis Ltd, Edinburgh
Cover printed by Clays Ltd, St Ives plc

ACKNOWLEDGEMENTS

I would like to thank a number of people for their contribution to the writing of this book. Firstly, my wife, Ros for putting up with me; secondly, Helen Reilly for her total professionalism and for getting the project up and running; and last, but no means least, all those poachers turned game-keepers for giving me the necessary inspiration!

Contents

Day-by-day guide to the secrets of Dr Mark Porter's Complete Lifeplan

INTRODUCTION

We all want to live life to the full and that's what this book's all about. It contains no fads, no quick fixes...no pointless reassurances. Instead, what I have tried to do is to come up with good, informative, well-researched advice that will enable you to make your own decisions about what you can do to improve your health and enhance your life.

As I do in my weekly *Radio Times* column, I have chosen subjects which reflect the problems I most commonly come across in my surgery and in my work as a radio and TV doctor. I have then looked for ways we can all most easily and effortlessly bring about changes for the good.

And I mean easily and effortlessly. We are all — doctors more than most — bombarded with advice on diet and exercise. Much of it is unrealistic and over-ambitious, so it is either ignored or leaves people thinking that they have to go the whole hog straight away. The couch potato buys some stretchy kit and starts going to the gym three times a week: six weeks later, bored, disillusioned and often injured, he/she gives up, never to return. Likewise, replacing chips, butter and bacon sandwiches with lentils and bran might be healthy but, yuk, for many of us it would be purgatory and very short-lived.

The whole idea of the book is that you do NOT have to do these sorts of things to be healthier and happier. What I say, instead, is that any step in the right direction is worth taking, whether it is cutting down on cigarettes or eating an extra piece of fruit a day.

Life is for living and enjoying. There's no point doing things just because they're healthy, we should do them because they are enjoyable and healthy, and it's okay to take the unhealthy option once in a while. To my mind, moderation never killed anybody, while gloomily taking the healthiest option at every turn would make the longer life achieved as a result inter-minable.

I've organised the book by days of the week – rather like *Radio Times* – not because you must do any one thing on a particular day, but because it's useful to have a thought for the day; a reminder of the area of your lifestyle to which you could pay some attention. The start of each 'day' also has a useful list of easy life-improvers because all I want to do is increase under-standing of the various aspects of life where we can most readily bring about changes for the good. If I succeed in this, I will be happy and hopefully you will be healthier and happier, too.

CHAPTER ONE

'WOW, I'LL NEVER NEED TO DIET AGAIN!'

★ **Cut down on all fats.**

★ **Eat at least five portions of fresh fruit and vegetables a day.**

★ **Replace some meat meals with fish.**

★ **Eat more carbohydrates, such as potatoes, wholemeal rice, pasta and bread.**

★ **Cut back on sweets and sugar.**

★ **Cut back on salt.**

★ **Get to know about essential vitamins and minerals (good for you) and TFAs (bad for you).**

SATURDAY'S CHOICE

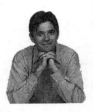

Eat Well

The healthy eating message has been falling on deaf ears for as long as I have been in general practice. The main problem, until very recently, was that nutritionists were not speaking in a language that the rest of us could understand. Even more to the point, the advice was not presented in a practical way that made healthy eating possible for the majority of us.

We are not all going to turn into lentil-eating vegetarians and I, for one, would think it a shame if we did.

Another reason is that, in 1994–5, the Health Education Authority spent £104 000 on nutritional education compared with £559 million spent by food manufacturers advertising mainly confectionery, soft drinks and fast foods. Given this disparity, it is hardly surprising that the healthy eating message is not getting through.

Time and time again, however, research shows that people do want to eat healthily, but confusion reigns about how to go about it. (To get off to a good start, see my fourteen-day healthy-eating meal plan guide, page 56.)

The healthy eating message also has to be realistic. We are not all going to turn into lentil-eating vegetarians and I, for one, would think it a shame if we did. At the same time, however, I have to admit that the link between our Western diet and many diseases is undeniable. Illnesses which can be laid at the door of our diet include heart disease, diabetes, high blood pressure, bowel cancer, constipation (we in the West spend an amazing sum supporting a laxative industry which is practically non-existent elsewhere), piles, tooth decay and gallstones.

Latest figures also show we are getting fatter and fatter with over half the adult population now overweight. This is a growing problem in every sense of the word. Overweight is defined as being ten per cent or more over the upper limit of our ideal weight. Obesity is when we are more than twenty per cent over our ideal weight (see page 43).

In a nutshell, the average Brit is eating too much fat, salt and sugar, and not enough starchy carbohydrates, fresh fruit and vegetables. Much of this is due to our reliance on processed foods – so-called 'convenience' foods out of a packet or can.

But there are no such things as 'bad' foods; only bad diets. A cream cake, for example, is not necessarily a 'bad' thing as long as it does not become a daily habit and make up a disproportionate amount of the food that we eat. It is more the way we balance the food we eat than the individual components themselves that cause problems. In other words, we can have a perfectly healthy diet that contains some so-called 'unhealthy foods' — occasional treats. The key is variety and moderation. If we stick to these principles, we will not go far wrong.

Fats

When it comes to healthy eating messages, advice about which fats we should be eating tops the list for confusion and misunderstanding. For this reason, I am going to keep the whys and wherefores to a minimum and concentrate instead on the practical aspects of a healthy eating diet. Fat is a vital building block for the body and an important source of energy. The problem arises when we eat too much of it. In the average British diet, fat makes up forty-two per cent of our daily calorific intake and, without doubt, this is the reason for our high rates of obesity. It is also a problem because we eat such high amounts of the wrong sorts of fat — the reason for our high rates of heart disease.

Rates of coronary heart disease

One in three men and one in four women die from coronary heart disease in this country, making it the leading cause of death in the UK, responsible for an annual death toll of 170 000 people. The problem is particularly serious in Scotland and Northern Ireland, both of which top the international heart disease league. There are a number of different factors, such as genetic predisposition and smoking habits, that explain this high incidence, but the principal one is almost certainly poor diet — in particular a very high intake of saturated fats.

In Southern European countries, such as France, Spain and Italy, where olive oil (monounsaturated fat) features so prominently in their diet the death rates are much lower — which is why doctors use the Mediterranean diet as a model for a healthy diet.

Within two years of reducing fat intake, there is a noticeable reduction in risk of heart disease and the full benefits are apparent in just five years.

The latest figures for death rates from coronary heart disease per 100 000 population are:

	Men	Women
Scotland	535	218
Northern Ireland	514	202
Ireland	490	161
Finland	479	135
Wales	445	171
England	409	154
USA	317	128
Australia	286	111
The Netherlands	267	87
Greece	212	63
Italy	184	56
Portugal	164	57
Spain	152	45
France	121	31
Japan	49	20

Health of the Nation targets

The Government's Health of the Nation campaign to reduce deaths from heart disease and stroke by at least forty per cent by the year 2000 has come up with the following target:

▶ Reduce your total calorie intake from fat from forty-two per cent to thirty-five per cent, and from saturated fat from sixteen per cent to eleven per cent. For the average British person this will mean cutting total fat consumption by 15 g (1 tablespoon) a day, and saturated fat intake by 11 g (2 teaspoons) a day (see Practicalities, page 22). ◀

There is a wealth of evidence testifying to the health benefits of these reductions (see Cholesterol – the facts, below). For example, in February 1994, doctors collected and analysed all the trials that investigated the relationship between fat and heart disease. What they discovered was that reducing fats in a diet to the recommended levels halves the likelihood of heart disease for a typical forty-year-old. It is also now known that the benefits take effect surprisingly quickly. Within two years of reducing fat intake, there is a noticeable reduction in risk and the full benefits are apparent in just five years.

Cholesterol – the facts

The link between fat and heart disease is cholesterol. But it is important to add that, despite its constant bad press, cholesterol is also a vital nutrient for the smooth running of the body. It is an essential component of cell membranes and is also needed to make a number of hormones, including oestrogen and testosterone.

The danger to health only arises when we have too much: the higher the level of cholesterol, the higher the risk of coronary disease. In Britain six out of ten adults have raised levels of cholesterol – that is above 5.2 mmol/l. The risk of heart disease then doubles for every ten per cent rise above this figure.

This risk is further raised when high levels are combined with other risk factors for heart disease – namely smoking, obesity, high blood pressure, a family history of heart disease and diabetes – all of which are common in this country.

This brings us to a controversial issue. Should everyone have a routine test to find out whether they are at increased risk? At the moment anybody who has any of the above-mentioned risk factors will probably be offered a test by their GP. Anyone can request a free test, but there seems to me little point in finding out that the level is too high, unless you intend to do something about your diet. If not, the chances are you will just worry yourself to death.

My own cholesterol level is too high – about 6.00 mmol/l – and I put this down to my fondness for cheese. Fortunately, as I don't smoke (any more) and I am pretty thin and fairly active, I am not unduly concerned. However, if the other factors were also in play then I would certainly do more to reduce my cholesterol level.

Home-testing cholesterol kits are pretty accurate and are now widely available but, for two reasons, I feel most people would be wiser to see their doctor. Firstly, as I have already mentioned, over half of the people who do these home tests will find that their cholesterol level is too high and will need to consult their doctor to find out what they should do about it. The first thing the doctor will do is retest. Secondly, in women the absolute cholesterol level may not be as important as the different types of cholesterol which occur in the blood known as HDL and LDL (see below). This can only be established by a GP test. So, you might as well cut out the middle man and go straight to your doctor.

HDL is the 'good' form of cholesterol because it is not deposited on the blood vessel walls and, in fact, appears to encourage the transfer of cholesterol back into the bloodstream therefore hindering the production of health-threatening fatty plaques which cause the arteries to fur up and narrow.

LDL is the 'bad' form – the type which ends up being deposited on the inner walls of the arteries where, as early as our late teens, it forms tiny fatty streaks. In time, these streaks can build up into fatty plaques, first reducing then possibly blocking the blood supply to vital organs such as the brain and the heart. This process, called atherosclerosis, makes heart attacks and strokes more likely. This tends to worsen with age, but there is some evidence to suggest that very low fat diets can, over a period of time, partly reverse this process.

In summary, if you have a high cholesterol level but a higher than average HDL to LDL ratio, then it is of less concern.

Before the menopause, women usually have higher levels of HDL. After the menopause, however, women produce much lower levels of the female hormone oestrogen which, in turn, leads to a shift in the balance of HDL and LDL. At this time HDL levels tend to drop and LDL levels rise. This is one of the reasons why women's risk of heart disease is so much higher after the menopause. Hormone replacement therapy (HRT) helps to counteract this effect and can reduce the risk of heart disease in post-menopausal women by as much as forty per cent.

A change of diet can reduce cholesterol levels by ten per cent. When this is also combined with exercise and, if necessary, weight loss, the reduction can be as much as twenty per cent. However, for patients with very high levels of cholesterol these reductions are not enough and special cholesterol lowering drugs will need to be prescribed.

Saturated fats

Saturated fats are one of three main types of fats, and are the ones which are associated with high levels of heart disease. These fats, usually of animal origin and found in dairy, meat and confectionery products, are very popular in Britain. We should all try to reduce our intake of this kind of fat and substitute, where necessary, with the other two types – monounsaturated and polyunsaturated.

Monounsaturated fats

Monounsaturated fats, such as olive and rapeseed oil, are the staple fats of Mediterranean countries which have significantly lower levels of heart disease than we do, even though they smoke and drink more.

Polyunsaturated fats

Polyunsaturated fats, such as vegetable oils, while better for us than saturated fats may not be as beneficial as monounsaturated. Marine fish oils are an exception and offer some protection against heart disease. (See below.)

Saturated fats

▶ Usually of animal origin: full-fat dairy products (whole milk, butter, hard cheeses, cream, ice-cream), meat with fat on it, meat products (for example, sausages, pasties and pies), confectionery, such as cakes, biscuits and chocolate, and fried food. The only vegetable oils which contain significant amounts of saturated fat are coconut and palm oil.

▶ They are not essential for a healthy diet: their only role is to provide energy or be deposited as fat.

▶ They raise LDL cholesterol (see Cholesterol – the facts, page 14) and a high intake is related to heart disease.

▶ Generally solid at room temperature.

Polyunsaturated fats

▶ Found mainly in oily fish, nuts and vegetable oils, such as corn oil and sunflower oil.

▶ Two forms of this fat are required in a healthy diet because they cannot be produced by the body – these are linoleic and alpha-linolenic acids which have become known as essential fatty acids.

▶ Some types have a favourable effect on blood cholesterol levels because they lower LDL (see Cholesterol – the facts, page 14). Even so, in excessive amounts, they are not beneficial.

▶ Generally liquid at room temperature.

Monounsaturated fats

▶ The richest sources are olive oil and rapeseed oil, but they are also found in peanuts and avocado pears.

▶ Until recently they were thought to have a neutral effect on cholesterol levels, but new research has shown that they can also lower LDL cholesterol (see pages 15–16).

▶ Usually liquid at room temperature.

Putting sound principles into practice

So now we know why we are supposed to be reducing saturated and polyunsaturated fats in favour of monounsaturated fats, how do we put good healthy-eating principles into practice? First, we need to know where fats are to be found in our diet. The following fat percentage chart will help to establish this.

Fat percentage	Product
	Meat and meat products
25 per cent	Butter and margarine
21 per cent	Cooking oils and fats
14 per cent	Milk
11 per cent	Cheese, and cream
7 per cent	Biscuits, cakes and pastries
7 per cent	Other foods
15 per cent	

Meats and meat products

Although about a quarter of the fat we eat comes from meat and meat products, the actual fat content varies tremendously within this group. So, it is necessary to consider the entire range, and then be more selective about what kind of meat and meat products you include in your diet. The following list will help you to do this. (See also Knowing your meat and fish, opposite.)

▶ The worst culprits in the fat stakes are meat products, such as sausages, pâtés or pasties. For example, up to a third of the calories in the average meat pie come from fat, and the average Brit eats seven portions of these products a week. Ideally, this should be halved.

▶ The latest Government recommendations do not call for a change in the amount of carcass meats we eat, but do suggest a switch towards lean meat. This could reduce total fat intake by about 3 g (½ a teaspoon) a day and saturates by just under 2 g a day.

▶ Eat more meats from the low-fat category instead of those from the high-fat category. Chicken or turkey – provided you do not eat the skin which is high in fat – are good options. Substitute fish for some meat meals.

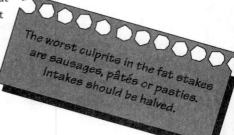

The worst culprits in the fat stakes are sausages, pâtés or pasties. Intakes should be halved.

KNOWING YOUR MEAT AND FISH

(see also Benefits of fish, page 24)

Low-fat meat: roast chicken and turkey (without skin); lean roast beef; venison and other game.

Medium-fat meat: lean boiled ham; lean roast duck (without skin); stewed offal; lean grilled pork chop; stewed rabbit; lean beef.

Medium- to high-fat meat: bacon; mince; chops; gammon; liver sausage; salami; luncheon meat; meat pies; pâtés; scotch eggs.

Low-fat fish: white fish (poached or steamed); canned fish in brine or water; prawns; scallops; trout (grilled or steamed).

Medium-fat fish: salmon, mackerel, herring, sardines and pilchards in tomato sauce.

Yellow spreads

Confusion also reigns when it comes to yellow spreads – butter and margarine. The first point is that butter and margarine contain the same number of calories and the same amount of fat, but differ in the type of fat.

Butter is high in saturated fats but relatively low in trans fatty acids (TFAs) (see What are trans fatty acids? page 20).

Margarine is low in saturated fats, but high in TFAs. It is also important to note that margarine labelled 'high in polyunsaturates' contains even lower amounts of saturated fatty acids than other margarines, but often greater amounts of TFAs. Given what we now know about TFAs, this means there is very little to choose between the two.

There really is no need to get too bogged down in all these details. The most important thing is to use all of them sparingly. If you do this, you do not need to worry about which you use and can choose the one you like.

WHAT ARE TRANS FATTY ACIDS (TFAs)?

The 1980s saw a big switch from butter to margarine mainly as a result of concern over saturated fats.

Margarine was portrayed by its manufacturers as the much healthier alternative to butter. Most of us duly switched. However, the bubble burst when people realised the potential risk of substances called trans fatty acids (TFAs) in margarine.

As I have already explained, polyunsaturated fats are liquid at room temperature and hence were no alternative to butter because they couldn't be spread. To get round this, manufacturers add TFAs which help to solidify fat. TFAs are produced by a process called hydrogenation and often appear in the list of ingredients as hydrogenated oils.

Some research, however, suggests they may have the same – or even worse – effect on the heart as saturated fats. One American nutritionist, Professor Walter Willett, claims TFAs may be to blame for 30 000 extra deaths a year from heart disease. He – supported by others – even attributes their introduction, earlier on in this century, with the current epidemic of heart disease.

Margarine and other non-butter spreads are the main source of these artificial fats, but they are also present in meat pies and other meat products, biscuits, cakes, buns and pastries. Fast food is another major source because it is often deep fried in partially hydrogenated oils.

Cooking oils: the main liquid vegetable oils in the UK are soy bean, rapeseed, sunflower, olive, peanut, safflower and corn oils. Blended oils are usually a mixture of soy bean and rapeseed oil. All these liquids can be used in cooking and salad dressings without too many worries because they are low in saturated fats and free from trans fatty acids. However, as they are still fats and are high in calories, it makes sense to use them sparingly.

Solid fats: the main solid fats used in the UK are animal based fats, such as butter, lard, dripping and, occasionally, palm and coconut oil – all of which are high in saturated fats. Specialised fats, made for baking and deep frying, are often made from partially hydrogenated vegetable oils. So, although they contain fewer saturated fats, they have higher amounts of TFAs. The best rule is to avoid solid fats whenever possible, but, if you have to use them, palm oil is probably the best.

HOW YOU CAN STILL FRY

Grilling and baking are by far the healthiest ways to cook. However, you do not have to throw away the frying pan – I certainly have not – you have to find ways to fry food without drenching it in fat.

★ First, make sure you have a good non-stick frying pan which means you do not need a lot of fat to fry in.

★ Always make sure you add the minimum of fat you need and pour away any excess. Avoid using solid fats, such as butter and lard, whenever possible.

★ Some foods can be fried without adding any fat because they contain enough fat to fry themselves – for example, minced meat, sausages and bacon. Other foods, instead of being cooked in copious amounts of pan oil, can just be brushed lightly with oil before frying.

★ Use kitchen roll to soak up any excess fat remaining on food after cooking.

Milk and other dairy products

Another big source of fat. Given what we now know about the dangers of a high-fat diet, there is no excuse for not using some low-fat dairy products.

Milk: skimmed milk contains virtually no fat but retains most of the nutritional benefits of full-fat milk. Likewise, semi-skimmed is preferable to full-fat. Low-fat milks should not be used for babies and children under three years because they need the additional calories in full-fat milk.

Cream: is particularly high in fat. Double cream contains forty-four per cent fat, single cream eighteen per cent. Low-fat versions are now available and other low-fat alternatives – especially useful for cooking but also as toppings – include low-fat natural yoghurt and low-fat fromage frais.

Cheese: is another rich source of fats and I am more than a little fond of

To date almost 130 research studies show a link between fresh produce and protection against cancer.

mine. However, even for me, it is certainly no hardship to use a low-fat cheese, such as Edam or a low-fat Cheddar in cooking. I certainly eat high-fat cheeses less often, and in much smaller portions. Because of the great variety of cheese now available, it makes sense to read the label carefully and to compare the fat content before deciding which ones to choose.

Biscuits, cakes, pastries and chocolate

Latest official recommendations suggest we should be halving our intake of cakes and biscuits – at the moment we eat an average of three to four biscuits a day. Chocolate should be reduced from a small bar (135 g/4¾ oz) each week to about three-quarters of a bar each week. This advice may seem harsh, but it is essential for all of us to appreciate the high fat content of these foods.

Food labelling

Good food labelling is making it easier to detect hidden fats and, in particular, the levels of saturated fats in foods. However, do bear in mind that some labelling can be misleading because it gives a percentage of the fat that the food contains. This is not a percentage of the number of calories present in the product because 1 g of fat contains more calories than the same amount of protein or carbohydrate.

Also, watch out for ambiguous labels that use meaningless terms such as reduced or virtually fat free. Generally speaking a food is only a low-fat food if it has less than 5 g/100 g fat present i.e. 5 g fat for every 100 g of the product.

The World Health Organisation recommend that adults should aim to eat about 500g (1 lb) of fruit and vegetables a day.

Practicalities

It's easy, then, to see how making small changes to our diet can help to meet the recommendations on fat intake. See table opposite for practical ideas.

We should be cutting our average consumption of total fat by 15 g (1 tablespoon) a day and 11 g (2 teaspoons) a day for saturated fat. Here is an indication of how these savings can easily be made.

Food swap	Total fat saving (grams)	Saturated fat saving (grams)
1 bowl of breakfast cereal with skimmed milk instead of whole milk	4	2
1 boiled egg instead of egg fried in oil	3	1
Reduced-fat Cheddar sandwich with low-fat spread instead of butter	19	15
1 banana instead of 2 digestive biscuits	7	3
1 apple instead of chocolate bar	15	9
2 grilled low-fat sausages instead of ordinary sausages	13	5
1 packet low-fat crisps instead of ordinary crisps	5	1
Pork chop – lean meat only instead of one with lean and fat	19	7
Steamed or boiled white fish instead of fish battered and fried in oil	33	3
Baked potato with cottage cheese instead of one with Cheddar topping	16	10

Benefits of fish

An Eskimo's staple diet is fish and it was the low rates of heart disease in Eskimos – they do not even have a word for heart disease in their vocabulary – that first drew nutritionists' attention to the dietary benefits of fish.

Fish is a rich source of protein and eating more of it – substituting it on occasions for meat – reduces the amount of saturated fats we eat. White fish – cod, haddock and plaice – are particularly low in calories and fat.

The main health benefits, however, are to be had from increasing our intake of oily fish, such as sardines, pilchards, herrings, mackerel, fresh (not canned) tuna, and salmon. Although these fish contain the same amount of fat as an average portion of meat – so you will not reduce your total fat consumption – the fat is predominantly unsaturated. More importantly they contain fats known as Omega-3 fatty acids which protect us against heart disease by lowering the levels of fat in the blood and making blood less likely to clot. It is these acids that are thought to be the reason why Eskimos have such a low incidence of heart disease. (NB: Canned fish is processed which means it loses a high percentage of Omega-3 fatty acids.)

Since various studies have shown that an increase of Omega-3 fatty acids in our diet can nearly halve the risk of heart disease, the Department of Health has responded to this evidence by recommending we eat about two portions of oily fish a week.

If you do not like fish you can take Omega-3 as a supplement. It is important, however, to buy this as capsules because in liquid form the Omega-3 content starts to reduce the moment the bottle is opened.

Fibre foods

Fibre was the big dietary story of the 1980s, when it was referred to as roughage, but it now seems to have lost its high-profile position partly because of the shift of interest to cholesterol. Nevertheless fibre plays a very important part in a healthy eating diet.

Dietary fibre is the indigestible part of plant foods. It has no nutritional value, but the bulk that it provides stimulates the muscular wall of the bowel allowing it to function more efficiently. In fact, it has a number of advantages. By helping to keep the bowel regular, conditions, such as constipation, bowel cancer, irritable bowel syndrome and piles, are reduced. These conditions, for example, are rare in countries where high fibre diets are the norm. In a fibre-rich diet, it takes twenty to fifty hours for food to travel the whole length of the gut. In the UK, as a direct result of the low fibre intake in the British diet, it takes on average around seventy hours and, in some cases, can take up to a week or ten days. As a result we are a nation of constipatees who spend over £40 million annually on laxatives.

The Department of Health advises us to eat around 18 g (¾ oz) of fibre a day. Unfortunately, our average consumption is nearer 9 g (⅜ oz).

High fibre diets have a number of other benefits, too, because they tend to be high in fresh produce and cereals, they also tend to be low in calories and fat – one of the reasons why Audrey Eyton's *F-plan Diet*, published by Penguin in 1982, became Britain's best-selling diet book of all time and was translated into sixteen languages. See adjacent list on how to increase the amount of fibre in your diet.

INCREASE FIBRE

★ Start the day with high-fibre breakfast cereal or muesli.

★ Eat two to four slices of wholemeal bread a day.

★ Include one of the following with your main meal – unpeeled potato, brown rice, wholemeal pasta or bulgar wheat.

★ Eat a portion of peas, beans or another pulse food, such as lentils, once a day.

★ In addition to the pulse family, eat at least one other fresh vegetable a day.

★ Eat two to five pieces of fresh fruit a day.

Fresh and frozen produce

In addition to containing a wide range of vitamins and minerals, fresh fruit and vegetables increase fibre in our diet and are low in calories.

To date almost 130 research studies show a link between fresh produce and protection against cancer – particularly cancer of the stomach and liver. One study showed that people who eat as little as one piece of fruit a day have half the risk of stomach cancer than those who eat none (see Foods that can protect against cancer, page 30).

In a 1990 report, the World Health Organisation recommended that adults should aim to eat about 500 g (1 lb) of fruit and vegetables a day, excluding potatoes. This amounts to approximately five servings a day. This is a very useful recommendation because it is concise and leaves no room for confusion. It can, however, be difficult to fulfil. Just consider how many portions you have had today. I bet these do not add up to the recommended five. So, a change of heart is needed.

Frozen foods are also good nutritional sources. In fact, some research shows that poor storage of fresh fruit and vegetables often means that their nutritional value is impaired or lost, while it can be retained in frozen foods because of the speed of processing. Fresh fruit and vegetables are most nutritious when eaten within two to three days of purchase and stored in chilled conditions. Tests of vitamin C content of fresh and frozen vegetables shows that frozen can be as good as fresh.

The main problem with fruit and vegetables is that it is only too easy to lose their nutritional benefits through poor cooking practices. However, it is possible to get round this (see box on left). Even so, it is always a good idea to eat them raw as often as possible.

Cooking tips

★ Cook vegetables and fruit for the shortest possible time.

★ Add them to boiling water and cook in the minimum amount of water.

★ Steaming and microwaving are better options than boiling.

★ Use the cooking water for soups and sauces. Cooking does not destroy nutrient-rich minerals, and they leach into the cooking water.

★ Always try and leave the skins on your fruit and vegetables whenever possible, but make sure you wash them thoroughly before cooking.

Salt

High levels of salt are responsible for raising blood pressure – which then increases our chances of heart disease and stroke. It is also linked with kidney stone formation, and some researchers believe that it plays a role in asthma. One study of asthmatic volunteers, for example, found that a high salt intake increases bronchial reactions – a major determinant in asthma attacks – and this finding is now under further investigation.

Other studies have linked a high salt intake with some cancers, particularly cancer of the stomach. Salt also plays a part in determining how much calcium is excreted from the body.

Our taste for salt in this country stems from the days when it was used as a preservative for meats and fish. With the advent of refrigeration salt was no longer needed, but by then we had got used to the taste and it continues to appear on our tables. The problem is that salt is present in most processed foods and we continue to add it when we are cooking, or at the table. As a result we are now consuming far more salt than we need. Nutritionists say that we should reduce our daily intake by an average of about 9 g per day to about 5 g for women and 7 g for men. One teaspoon of salt equals 6.5 g.

The most obvious way to achieve this is to reduce, or preferably cut out, the habit of adding salt to food during cooking. But you will be surprised how little this helps. For example, boiling one portion of potatoes or peas in salted water compared to unsalted water saves only 0.3 g of salt in potatoes and 0.2 g salt in peas. The overall saving of not adding salt to food at home will only be about 1.5 g a day. The reason for this is that the main sources of salt in the UK diet – about eighty-five per cent – are manufactured canned foods, ready-made meals and bread. For example, one slice of bread contains 0.4 g salt. This means it requires effort from us to reduce this health hazard in our diet and, as the responsibility chiefly lies with manufacturers, it is another good reason for avoiding processed foods and increasing the use of fresh foods.

Reducing salt intake is of particular importance for people with high blood pressure, because salt reduction is one of the first line treatments that doctors try. For people who find food completely unappetising without salt, low sodium salt is a useful substitute.

Sugars vs unrefined carbohydrates

Carbohydrates can be divided into two main groups. Refined carbohydrates, such as sugar; and unrefined (starchy) carbohydrates, such as potato, rice, pasta and bread.

We eat far too much of the refined carbohydrates in the form of added sugar, cakes, biscuits, and confectionery. Sugars are not only fattening they can also worsen specific health problems, such as dental decay and diabetes.

In contrast, unrefined starchy carbohydrates provide an excellent source of energy with few if any medical risks and are the ideal ingredients for low-fat low-sugar diets.

Vegetarianism and veganism

The Vegetarian Society defines a vegetarian as somebody who does not eat flesh, fowl or fish and avoids by-products of slaughter, such as leather goods.

In addition there are some people who could be described as 'partial vegetarians'. This group eats fish and poultry, and uses by-products of slaughter, such as leather goods and lipstick.

A vegan is a vegetarian who, in addition to not eating flesh, fowl or fish, does not eat eggs or any dairy products, such as butter, milk and cheese.

Studies show that both vegetarians and vegans are motivated by three key factors:

▶ A respect for animals.
▶ Environmental awareness.
▶ The health implications of a meat-free diet.

There is no doubt that a good vegetarian diet is the healthiest diet we can have.

Vegetarianism is more than a fad. Numbers have swelled from 100 000 in 1945 to over three million today and the Vegetarian Society claims that another 2000 people join its ranks each week. There is no doubt that a good vegetarian diet is the healthiest diet we can have. Many studies testify to this. The most recent study followed up over 11 000 meat-eaters and vegetarians in Oxford and found that vegetarianism had cut the death rate from heart disease by twenty-eight per cent and cancer by thirty-nine per cent.

However, the study's author, Dr Margaret Thorogood of the London School of Hygiene and Tropical Medicine, who is herself a meat-eater, stressed that the results do not provide justification for immediately giving up meat. Although this may seem illogical, there is no scientific evidence as yet that meat is the reason for more deaths among meat-eaters. The differences could be due to other factors in the diet, such as a vegetarian diet tends to be higher in fresh produce, fibre and starchy carbohydrates and antioxidants, and lower in saturated fats and calories, as well as differences in lifestyle. Studies show that vegetarians are more likely to be non-smokers, more moderate alcohol drinkers, and more likely to appreciate the benefits of a healthy diet.

My advice is eat meat, if you want to, but make sure you supplement it with lots of vegetables and fruit. In my view, it really comes down to personal taste – our bodies can do without meat, but eaten in moderation it does us no harm.

Converting to vegetarianism

If this is on your mind, remember that a healthy vegetarian diet involves a lot more than suddenly cutting out meat from your diet. You will need to learn as much as possible about your nutritional requirements and how to ensure that you are getting them. Here is what you should look out for:

Energy: this can be easily met by a vegetarian diet, but be aware that diets composed primarily of fruit and vegetables are bulky, making it sometimes difficult to eat enough of them to meet your energy requirements. Children, in particular, find vegetarian diets very filling and may find it difficult to eat enough calories at each meal. Useful energy-rich vegetarian additions include nuts and seeds and foods cooked with vegetable oils.

Protein: in the past most concerns about a vegetarian diet centred on possible shortages of protein. The protein intake of vegetarians is slightly lower than that of non-vegetarians, but still meets the current UK dietary recommendations and is unlikely to have any detrimental effect. Useful vegetarian sources of protein include cereals, nuts and pulses such as beans and lentils.

Fats: the total fat intake of vegetarians and meat eaters is usually similar. In vegans the fat intake is healthily lower. This is because, unlike meat eaters and vegetarians, vegans do not eat dairy products. All vegetarians and vegans have the major advantage of having a lower intake of saturated fats than meat eaters, and this can be as low as five per cent in vegans.

Carbohydrates: many studies confirm minimal differences in total intake of carbohydrates between meat eaters and vegetarians.

Foods that can protect against cancer

Epidemiologists believe that as many as one in three cancers are caused by dietary factors – and the figure could be much higher than this for certain cancers. In particular, many of the studies suggest that a diet rich in vegetables and fruit protects us against cancer of the stomach, oesophagus, large bowel and lung. Most of these studies looked at the amount of fruit and vegetables included in the diet of various populations and compared this with their cancer rates.

It remains uncertain precisely what it is in fruit and vegetables that is responsible for this protective effect. To date, most of the attention has been paid to antioxidant vitamins (see Antioxidants and free radicals, page 34), but it is still unproven whether these increase the protection.

For example, one study, known as the Linxian Intervention Study, involved giving the antioxidant vitamins E, beta carotene and vitamin C to a population in North Central China. Characteristically, this population has a low vitamin and mineral intake and a very high cancer rate, particularly of the stomach and oesophagus. The result of the antioxidant supplements experiment showed a twenty per cent reduction in mortality from cancers after just over five years.

Other results, however, are contradictory. Finnish researchers tried to replicate the effect of fruit and vegetables by giving vitamin supplements to a group of male smokers in the hope that it would reduce cancer – particularly lung cancer – mortality. The disappointing results suggested that among the new cases of lung cancer, those who had received the antioxidant, beta carotene, were actually at increased risk of lung, bladder and stomach cancers, a finding backed by an even larger study in America.

These results serve to reinforce the point that scientists and doctors do not really know what it is in fruit and vegetables that protects us against cancer. It may indeed be the antioxidants, but they may need to be taken with other substances which occur naturally in fruit and vegetables, but are not included in the many supplements. Or it may be due to the high fibre content of these foods. We know, for example, that fibre reduces the risk of bowel cancer. Likewise, it may be that eating lots of fruit and vegetables tends to lower people's intake of other harmful nutrients, such as salt and saturated fat.

All these possibilities – and the role of other foods – are still under investigation in a massive study called the European Prospective Investigation of Cancer (EPIC). In this, some 400 000 participants from seven countries, including the UK, are being recruited and monitored for the next ten years.

In the meantime, the best advice is to include lots of fruit and vegetables in your diet because, at the moment, we know of no better substitute for this.

VITAMINS

Vitamin A: an essential building block for pigments in the eye. Lack of vitamin A can cause night blindness. The richest dietary source is retinol in animal foods and carotenoids from pigmented foods and vegetables. The higher intake of the latter usually makes up for any shortfall of retinol in a vegetarian diet.

B vitamins: these have a wide range of functions and a deficiency can lead to neurological problems, such as a loss of physical sensation, weakness and anaemia. Riboflavin and vitamin B12 are typically found in meat, fish and dairy products, so vegans need to watch out for a shortfall in this one. Having said that, good vegetarian sources include breakfast cereals, Marmite and Vecon vegetable stock.

Vitamin C: this vitamin, like vitamin E below, is an important antioxidant (see opposite and page 34) and is usually found in higher quantities in a vegetarian diet. Vitamin C is needed for the production of collagen – the main structural protein in the skin. A deficiency leads to scurvy.

Vitamin D: this is needed for healthy bones and a deficiency can lead to rickets. Its dietary sources are usually animal (which is why vegetarians can lack it). It is present in many fortified foods, especially margarine (but see section on TFAs on page 20). Vegetarians and vegans may need to compensate for a lack of vitamin D by dietary supplements in late winter and early spring.

Vitamin E: like vitamin C, above, this is an important antioxidant (see opposite and page 34) and is usually found in higher quantities in a vegetarian diet. It is needed to protect cell walls. A deficiency can cause mild anaemia and neurological problems such as loss of balance.

KEY MINERALS

Iron: this is a key component of haemoglobin – the pigment contained in red blood cells which carries oxygen from the lungs to the muscles and tissues of the body. Vegetarians are no more likely to lack it than meat-eaters. Ensuring sufficient intake of it is particularly important for babies and toddlers (see Vitamin and mineral supplements, opposite) and women – and even meat-eaters can be at risk of anaemia. Good non-meat sources of iron include leafy green vegetables, pulses (including baked beans), dried fruit, wholemeal bread and fortified breakfast cereals.

Calcium: over ninety-nine per cent of the body's calcium is contained in the skeleton. The remaining one per cent performs many vital functions including helping blood to clot and muscles to contract. Most of the calcium in an ordinary diet comes from milk and cheese, so low calcium intake can be a problem for vegans, and, left unchecked, may predispose them to osteoporosis later in life. A calcium supplement may also be necessary for teenagers and breast feeding mothers.

Daily vitamin recommendations for vegetarians

The Vegetarian Society recommends that a vegetarian diet should include the following:

★ Three to four servings of cereals/grains – to provide energy, fibre, vitamin B, calcium and iron.

★ Two to three servings of pulses, nuts or seeds – to provide protein, energy, fibre, calcium, iron and zinc.

★ Four to five servings of fruit and vegetables, including dark green leafy vegetables (folate or folic acid, calcium and iron), red, orange and yellow vegetables (beta-carotene), fresh fruit for vitamin C, and dried fruit to provide fibre and iron.

★ Two servings of dairy or soya products – to provide proteins, energy, calcium and other minerals, vitamin B12 and D.

★ A small amount of plant oils, margarine or butter – to provide energy, essential fatty acids, and vitamin E, A and D.

Vitamin and mineral supplements

The British spend more than £200 million a year on vitamin and mineral supplements and, for the most part, the money might as well be thrown down the drain. This is because it is no secret that supplements are most often taken by people who are least in need of them — that is those who are nutritionally aware and on the best diets anyway.

The main reason for taking supplements is to avoid basic vitamin or mineral deficiencies which is unlikely for most people in the Western world. I would only recommend them in the following situations:

▶ Some young children — particularly those under twelve months who are given cows' milk as their main drink, and those who are solely breastfed for longer than six months — may suffer from iron-deficiency anaemia. This is because cows' milk — and breast milk — are comparatively low in iron. Cows' milk should never be used instead of formula milk as a main drink for babies under twelve months. Formula milk is supplemented with iron and vitamins A, C and D. Some long-term breastfed babies may benefit from vitamin A, C, D and iron supplements. So, if you are considering breastfeeding for longer than six months, consult your GP. In October 1994, the British Nutrition Foundation called for urgent action to reduce the number of toddlers suffering from iron-deficiency anaemia.

▶ There is also growing evidence that a poor diet can increase the chances of behaviourial problems in children. A good multivitamin and mineral supplement is now thought to lessen the problem.

▶ Women trying to become pregnant should take folic acid before they try to conceive and up until the twelfth week of pregnancy. Studies have proved that this dramatically reduces the chances of the baby having spina bifida or related conditions.

▶ Those with special dietary needs, such as people with absorption problems or very restricted diets, may need supplements.

▶ Women, particularly those past menopause, and men with a high risk of osteoporosis can benefit from calcium and vitamin D supplements.

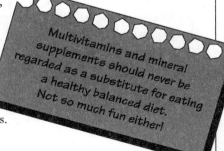

Multivitamins and mineral supplements should never be regarded as a substitute for eating a healthy balanced diet. Not so much fun either!

Eating the skins

There has been much recent concern about the levels of insecticide residues found in the skins of some vegetables. Most of the recent publicity has centred on carrots, which many people love to eat raw. In response to this anxiety about residual organophosphates used to control carrot fly, the Ministry of Agriculture, Fisheries and Food advised people to peel and top carrots before eating them. Not surprisingly, organically grown fruit and vegetables (grown without the use of any insecticides) have enjoyed a surge in popularity.

The controversy surrounding the use of insecticides and their possible effect on those at the end of the food chain – us – will doubtless continue for many years to come, but thoroughly washing vegetables is currently considered more than adequate protection for other produce.

Antioxidants and free radicals

Recently there has been heightened interest in the antioxidant vitamins which are vitamins C, E and beta-carotene (which is converted into vitamin A in the body). These are increasingly being taken in megadoses – levels far in excess of the recommended daily intake; typical examples of such high doses are 500–1000 mg vitamin C and 100–200 iu (international units) of vitamin E a day.

If the claims are to be believed, they can help us to live longer, look younger, halve our risk of cancer and heart disease, and protect us against all sorts of other conditions from cataracts to arthritis. True or false? Well, to be honest, the jury is still out and I, for one, remain to be convinced.

The theory goes that antioxidants work by scavenging and deactivating free radicals – the unstable and potentially damaging waste products of many bodily reactions. Free radicals are also produced by exposure to pollution, tobacco smoke and sunlight. They are known to damage cells by a process known as oxidation – which is easy to understand when you appreciate that oxidation of iron and steel is known as rusting.

Unwanted oxidation reactions occur all the time. For example, cooking oils go rancid, apples turn brown, uncorked wine goes vinegary. And just as we can prevent apples turning brown with lemon juice, the theory claims that we can prevent the damage wrought by free radicals by taking megadoses of antioxidants.

While this looks very promising on paper, the evidence is somewhat mixed and, as yet, too inconclusive for doctors to recommend them. Two recent studies have highlighted the possibility that high doses of antioxidants could actually be harmful. The first, a Finnish study of more than 29 000 smokers, showed that men who took beta-carotene for six years had a slightly higher incidence of lung cancer than others.

Such results highlight the need to find out more before any conclusions can be finalised and advice given. I welcome the fact that the Medical Research Council and the British Heart Foundation are currently recruiting around 20 000 people to take part in the trial which will hopefully answer the antioxidant question once and for all.

In the meantime, the best thing you can do is to make sure you maximise your intake of these vitamins by meeting the current recommendations for including fruit and vegetables in your diet, that is five portions of fruit and vegetables a day (see page 56).

GARLIC

There is growing evidence that eating large amounts of garlic can help protect us against heart disease and reduce high blood pressure. The active ingredient is a compound called allicin which is produced when garlic is cut or crushed. Unfortunately allicin is also the part of the garlic which is responsible for its characteristic smell which is excreted from the body via the lungs.

To get around this problem some manufacturers produce odour-free garlic capsules. But the only way garlic can be odour-free is if it contains no allicin, which means you would be wasting your time and money. What the manufacturers really mean is that they have packaged the capsules in such a way that they will not release the garlic until they are past the stomach. This may stop the garlic 'repeating', but will have little effect on your breath because the allicin is absorbed into the blood from where it travels to the lungs where it is excreted in your breath – which basically means smelly breath to some degree is inevitable. French chefs are reputed to overcome the problem by eating parsley stalks.

Food additives

Despite their constant bad press, food additives actually make food safer, keep longer and stop the growth of bacteria. They can even improve its nutrient value – vitamin E, for example, is a natural additive. There are nearly 4000 substances in Britain which can be used legally as additives – most are flavourings. These do not have to be specified on the label except in the most general terms. The use of all other additives is controlled by law and they have to be safe, effective and necessary to be included.

E numbers: in addition, all additives that have been approved by the European Union are given an E number. However, older additives such as salt and vinegar have slipped past this net because of their long record of safety.

Allergic reactions: additives pose no threat to the health of most of us, but a few people do have an adverse reaction to additives, such as benzoic acid E210 or tartrazine E102 (see table opposite).

The only justifiable objection that can be raised about additives is that they can be used to disguise poor-quality food.

What about the children?

Much concern is currently being voiced about children's fondness for junk food and confectionery. However, last year's Medical Research Council report, the National Diet and Nutrition Survey of Children, which resulted from studying 1500 under-five-year-olds, contained some good news. It revealed that the pre-school children it studied were, in general, eating well and had good intakes of essential nutrients. Indeed their diet probably explained why the average five-year-old in Britain is more than 2.5 cm (1 inch) taller than the 1960s' crop.

There is also growing evidence that a poor diet can increase the chances of behavioural problems in children.

Having said that, the survey also highlighted some deficiencies – most notably iron. One in four of the children studied had below the recommended levels and one in eight of the youngest age groups were anaemic. This is particularly worrying because there is mounting evidence that iron

E NUMBERS

Though additives in general do not cause problems, you may find there are some which do affect you or your family. One problem that may be additive-related is hyperactivity, otherwise known as Attention Deficit/Hyperactivity Disorder (ADHD) – a condition that affects as many as ten per cent of the population and can be particularly troublesome in children. Some of the symptoms in infants include:

★ crying, screaming, restlessness, little sleep
★ colic; very difficult to feed (breast or bottle)
★ excessive dribbling and thirst

Symptoms in older children include:

★ clumsiness, impulsiveness, proneness to accidents
★ erratic, disruptive behaviour
★ aggression
★ poor appetite
★ poor hand and eye co-ordination

If you are affected by this problem, contact the Hyperactive Children's Support Group (address at the end of the chapter) who suggest, among other measures, avoiding the following additives:

E102 Tartrazine
E104 Quinoline Yellow
E110 Sunset Yellow FCF
E122 Carmoisine or Azorubine
E123 Amaranth
E124 Ponceau 4R or Cochineal
E127 Erythrosine B5
E128 Red 2G
E129 Allura Red AC
E131 Patient Blue V
E132 Indigo carmine or Indigotine
E133 Brilliant Blue FCF
E142 Green S (Acid Brilliant Grn)

E150 Caramel (a),(b), (c) or (d)
E151 Black PN (Brilliant Black BN)
E153 Carbon Black (Vegetable carbon)
E154 Brown FK (kipper brown)
E155 Brown HT
E210 Benzoic Acid
E211 Sodium Benzoate
E250 Sodium Nitrite
E251 Sodium Nitrate
E252 Potassium Nitrate
E320 Butylated Hydroxy Anisole
E321 Butylated Hydroxy Toluene

Asthmatics and aspirin-sensitive people who experience a numbing of the mouth or skin reactions may find these symptoms are related to particular additives such as those between E212 and E228 inclusive.

deficiency influences mental development and classroom performance.

The main reason for the deficiency is parents' too early use of 'doorstep' milk (cows' milk) instead of powdered infant formula milk. Ordinary cows' milk is not a good source of iron whereas infant bottle-feeding formulae are fortified with iron.

Once a child is weaned, the most readily available food source of iron is meat. Vegetarian sources (see Vitamin recommendations for vegetarians, page 32) are also fine, provided the diet also includes fruit – and it usually does. This is because vitamin C doubles the rate of iron absorption. Also bear in mind that it is never a good idea to give young children tea to drink because the tannin this contains prevents the absorption of iron.

Other findings, highlighted by the Department of Health, emphasise the need to encourage children to eat more vegetables and fruit. In one study only fifty per cent of the children ate apples and pears; just under fifty per cent ate bananas; and only twenty-five per cent ate oranges and other citrus fruits.

So, while most children are getting the basic nutrients they need we can do a lot better. More emphasis needs to be placed on fresh produce (fruit and vegetables) – and the earlier it is introduced after weaning the better. It is never too early to start eating healthily.

WARNING TO PARENTS

Many of the healthy-eating messages we have discussed in this chapter apply to children – but some do not apply to babies and young ones under two years. Research at Surrey University shows that if parents apply low-fat diet and high-fibre diet principles to children under two years they can put their children's growth and development at risk. For example, breast milk contains as much as sixty per cent of its energy in the form of fat – a level that would have the rest of us heading to the cardiac ward – but essential for a baby's normal growth and development!

Having said that, all parents need to bear in mind that most of us pick up our lifelong dietary habits – good and bad – at a young age. So, if we set out to bring up children, over the age of two, on the healthy diet outlined here, it will have major advantages later in life.

Using diet to control weight

Dieting has never been more popular. Today more than a third of the people in this country – and more than half of all women – are on a diet. And there is very little people will not try if they think it will help them lose more weight quickly. The diet industry – worth £1 billion a year – is well aware of this and there is no end to its ingenuity when it comes to cashing in on people's worries about their weight.

Appetite suppressants, meal replacements, slimming patches, creams, body wraps, diuretics (water tablets) have all become very fashionable. And, if all else fails, there is always the plastic surgeon's knife and cosmetic surgery.

Despite all this, we are still a nation of fatties and, what is more, we are getting fatter. Working on the basis that a person is overweight when they are more than ten per cent above their ideal weight, and obese when more than twenty per cent over, nearly half of all men and a third of all women are overweight. In addition, one in seven women and one in eight men are obese – that is more than twice as many as six years ago.

Although, in many respects, the obsession with dieting has become unhealthy, the health risks of obesity make this a problem that cannot be dismissed, and one that the Government is targeting. So what are the answers?

WHY DIETING FAILS

It is not difficult to work out why so many diets fail. The problem is that while many can lead to short-term weight loss, this is rarely sustained. For the most part, as soon as a person achieves a certain weight loss and comes off a diet, the weight starts to pile back on again because most people return to their old eating habits – the very reason they were overweight in the first place!

At last, after endless failures, there is a growing awareness that the only way to lose weight and keep it off is not to diet. The real answer is to adopt a gradual and permanent change for the better in our eating habits. Dieting will soon hopefully be a *passé* word.

Your ideal weight

Although, in principle, I do not approve of the idea of aiming for a specific weight loss, I have included an 'ideal weight chart' (on page 44) because everybody expects them. This approach, however, is rapidly becoming outdated because, in truth, it is daft to suggest that everyone of a certain height should be a certain weight.

What is far more important is to concentrate on achieving a healthy diet and to be more active. If we do this, then we can be reasonably confident that our weight will be right for us. It is also important to remember that, from a health point of view – and particularly for women – plumpness can actually be beneficial. For example, osteoporosis – the bone thinning disease, and a major cause of pain, deformity and fractures in later life – is much more likely to affect thin women than plump women.

> More than a third of the people in the UK – and more than half of all women – are on a diet.

Weight charts

The first thing to say is, please, be very wary about the so-called ideal weight charts produced by some diet clubs and slimming organisations. They sometimes recommend weights that are far too low for your height, and this is not only unethical, it is dangerous. Charts like these may encourage men and women to aim for a body weight that is unattainable through normal dieting and may cause the type of abnormal eating patterns that can lead to a full-blown eating disorder.

The weights given in the original charts were taken from a survey, conducted between 1935 and 1953, of nearly five million insurance policy holders in the United States. Since then, the charts have been adjusted upwards, but are still in my opinion on the low side. It is also important to remember that the original survey only considered how long people lived, and not how healthy or happy those years were. Quantity isn't always the same as quality.

Self-destructive dieting

Becoming obsessed with weight loss and trying to live up to the thin-as-a-plank role models can literally destroy lives. Today, this road to self-destruction, slow suicide, can begin very young. In a recent survey, which studied 50 000 schoolchildren, six out of ten sixteen-year-olds thought they were too fat; four in five fifteen-year-olds said their weight was a constant source of worry; and one in five admitted to 'skipping' meals in order to keep slim.

The problem is not confined to girls. It is a growing problem for boys, too. There are even reports that children – boys and girls as young as five – are starting to worry about their weight. Such findings are certainly reflected in the increase of eating disorders, such as anorexia nervosa, when a person can literally starve him or herself to death, and bulimia, when a person binges and then make themselves vomit.

From an adult point of view, it is also important to accept that weight gain is an inevitable consequence of getting older and that trying to fight what is reasonable and natural can be harmful. Health is not a question of being as slim as possible – far from it. In reality, there is a fine balance, and being too slim can be as unhealthy – or even unhealthier – than being too fat. This aspect is all too commonly forgotten.

As Mary Evans Young, founder of Dietbreakers and the international No Diet Day, said: 'I am not suggesting that every person who diets can end up with an eating disorder, but every person with an eating disorder started out as a person who was dieting.'

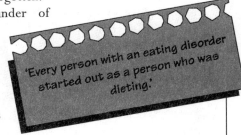

'Every person with an eating disorder started out as a person who was dieting.'

Are you really overweight?

Working out your ideal weight, while taking into consideration the different shapes and sizes, is not easy. In 1995, Scottish researchers decided to get around this problem by studying whether just one measurement – that of a person's waist circumference – could be used instead. They then came up with the following guidelines for men and women:

▶ Men with a waist circumference of between 94–102 cm (37–40 in), and women between 80–88 cm (31–35 in), are borderline overweight cases who should be careful not to put on any more weight. Obviously the younger a person is, the more potentially serious is the problem.

▶ Men with a waist measurement equal to or greater than 102 cm (40 in), and women greater than 88 cm (35 in), are appreciably overweight and should make efforts to lose weight. These measurements correspond with obesity-related health problems, such as breathlessness and arthritis.

It is not just total bodily fat that is important in determining weight-related health problems – such as heart disease – but where the fat is actually stored in the body can make a big difference.

There are two main body shapes. Apples who have most of their fat laid down around their waist and tummy, and pears who have most of the fat on their bottom and thighs. Weight for weight, apples have a higher chance of health problems, particularly heart disease.

If you are not sure whether you are an apple or pear, then you can find out by working out your waist-hip ratio. For apples this is high, and for pears it is low. Try the following:

▶ Measure your waist and hips.

▶ Divide the waist measurement by the hip measurement to get the waist-hip ratio. For example, if your waist is 86 cm (34 in) and your hips 102 cm (40 in), your waist–hip ratio will be 86 divided by 102 = 0.85.

▶ The ratio should be less than 0.95 in men and less than 0.87 in women.

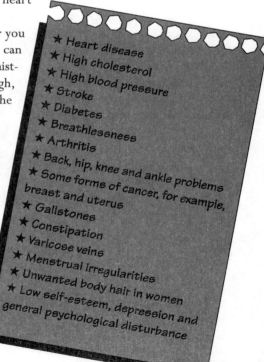

★ Heart disease
★ High cholesterol
★ High blood pressure
★ Stroke
★ Diabetes
★ Breathlessness
★ Arthritis
★ Back, hip, knee and ankle problems
★ Some forms of cancer, for example, breast and uterus
★ Gallstones
★ Constipation
★ Varicose veins
★ Menstrual irregularities
★ Unwanted body hair in women
★ Low self-esteem, depression and general psychological disturbance

Obesity – the health risks

Obesity is probably the single most common cause of ill health in the UK. Someone who is obese is up to twelve times more likely to die than someone of the same age of 'ideal' weight. Obviously the risks depend on how overweight the person is, but they start to rise significantly when the average man or women is more than 13 kg (2 stone) overweight.

Some of the health risks are due to specific metabolic changes in the body, such as high levels of cholesterol, others are simply due to the mechanical weight-bearing strain put on the various parts of the body. Most are interlinked. Recognised complications of being overweight are listed opposite.

Plump is good!

Do not confuse being at the upper end of your normal weight range, or even being slightly overweight, with being obese. There is increasing evidence to show that plumpness may be associated with some health benefits. Many doctors now argue that the so-called ideal weights, particularly those for women, are too low. Plump women, for instance, are less likely to have problems with fertility, give birth to bigger and healthier babies, and find breastfeeding easier.

Some recent studies have also suggested that both plump men and women stand a better chance of surviving a heart attack than people who are underweight.

UNDERWEIGHT – THE HEALTH RISKS

In many ways being underweight can be just as, if not more, dangerous than being overweight. Recognised health complications include:

★ Absent periods and infertility
★ Early menopause
★ Unwanted body hair
★ Osteoporosis
★ All consequences of malnutrition, including anaemia, muscle wastage and heart problems

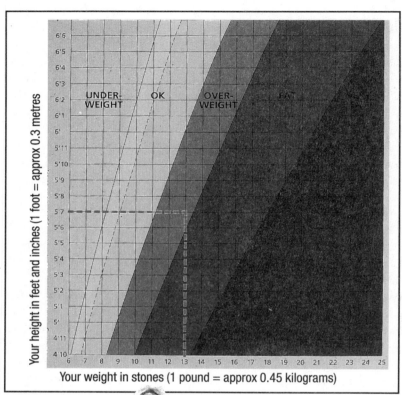

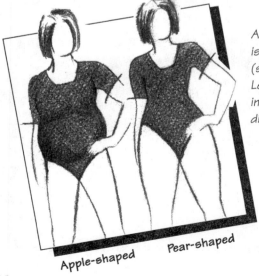

Apple-shaped   Pear-shaped

Above: this ideal weight chart is more generous than most (see page 40).
Left: where the fat is stored in the body can make a big difference.

Making excuses for why we get fat

It is very easy to blame weight problems on metabolism (the rate at which a body uses up the calories in food), and in the 1970s it was genuinely believed that slow metabolism was often the cause of overweight and obesity problems. However, recent research from Cambridge has shown that metabolic rate is rarely the cause of being fat. (See Basal metabolic rate (BMR), page 46.)

What was happening to confuse the issue in the 1970s was that obese people, who were claiming they ate less than their thin companions, were actually being economical with the truth. In actual fact they were eating far more than they claimed during the various studies and dotors, who were taken in by the claims, came up ever more frequently with the slow-metabolism theory.

It is very easy to blame weight problems on metabolism, but research shows this is rarely the cause.

Since the 1970s, the slow metabolism theory has proved very difficult to dispel and is now reflected in the intense interest shown in another theory – the obesity gene.

GLANDULAR PROBLEMS

A common misconception is that very overweight people have some kind of glandular problem that makes excessive weight gain inevitable. While, in theory, conditions such as an underactive thyroid can make people prone to weight gain, in practice this is rarely the cause. Only a tiny proportion of overweight people have an underlying medical condition that can be blamed. In most cases it is simply a matter of overeating!

I agree it would be nice if we could blame all our weight problems on our metabolic rate and genes, but today's rate of obesity is going up so fast that it is impossible to explain it all away with these two theories. I remain convinced – as do most nutritionists – that the chief reasons for being overweight are behavioural ones – overeating and too little activity. Sorry!

Basal metabolic rate (BMR)

This is the number of calories we burn up during periods of complete mental and physical rest – in other words when we are not doing anything. The figure for an average man is around 1800 calories a day. For the average woman it is about 1500. This rate is proportionately higher in young children, but falls as they get older.

Anxiety and tension both raise BMR, as do some hormonal conditions such as an overactive thyroid gland.

The BMR falls during periods of strict dieting, fasting or starvation, which explains why weight gain is more rapid in the first week or so after a diet while the BMR is readjusting.

Appetite control

Research shows that fat people tend to underestimate their food intake – on average by about 800 calories a day – the equivalent of three Mars bars or two cheese-and-ham sandwiches.

So what determines appetite? One way to understand why some people eat more than others is to consider the various influences that are at work before going on to consider the effect of different foods on appetite.

Appetite control is affected by many things – not just the type of food we eat, but also factors which determine when and how we eat. For example, just think how much more food we tend to eat at a buffet; or when we are with other people. How many times have you been persuaded to have a sticky toffee pudding when you would not normally consider one.

Mood also plays a part. Some people turn to food when they are feeling depressed, or stressed: so-called comfort-eating.

So, having dealt with the more subtle influences, let's move on to the different types of food and the growing understanding of how these influence appetite.

It is now generally accepted

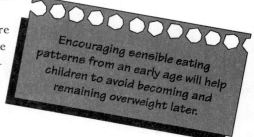

Encouraging sensible eating patterns from an early age will help children to avoid becoming and remaining overweight later.

that the main determining factor of whether we are hungry or not is the amount of carbohydrate, for example, bread, pasta and sugary foods, we have eaten. It appears that fatty foods, although high in calories, are not as good at satisfying our appetites as carbohydrates.

This is why a bread roll or piece of toast often fills a gap so much more effectively than a hunk of cheese. Refined or sugary carbohydrates, on the other hand, such as a bar of chocolate can 'kill' appetite by causing a rapid rise in blood sugar, but the effect is short-lived. This is because the rapid rise is soon followed by a precipitous fall, which once again 'triggers' hunger pangs. This is one reason why such foods are described as 'empty' calories.

The reason we have developed in this way may be due to evolutionary pressures. After all, if we consider traditional diets, fats were very scarce while carbohydrates, such as rice and potatoes, were the main source of energy. Perhaps as a direct result of this, our bodies developed a propensity for deciding when sufficient had been eaten by monitoring carbohydrate intake.

In the past, fats were certainly a rarity and therefore needed little or no regulation. When they were available, they were often stored for periods when other more common foodstuffs were hard to find.

Unfortunately our present diet could not be more different. Fats are now plentiful and account for over two-fifths of our daily calorie intake.

Genetic factors

Another important influence on eating habits is the influence that parents have on their children. It is certainly interesting to note that many children of overweight parents also end up being overweight themselves.

There are two possible explanations for this, both as yet poorly researched and understood. Firstly, due to hereditary factors, children may inherit a tendency to be overweight; secondly, they are very likely to be conditioned into adopting the eating habits of their parents – and continue to do so even when they are grown up. There is nothing that can be done about a genetic predisposition to being overweight, but much can be done about encouraging sensible eating patterns from an early age that will help children to avoid becoming and remaining overweight later in life – a little effort now could reap major benefits later in their lives.

MYTHS AND MISUNDERSTANDINGS

Dieting is steeped in more confusion and myth than most subjects: all our rationality seems to go out of the window! Or maybe it is just desperation – we would all like to believe that weight loss can be effortless, which is why so many of us are prepared to try new gimmicks even if reason tells us they are cons. So what are the commonest myths?

★ **If you have not stuck to the letter of your diet, then you might just as well give up.** The problem with many diets is that people assume they have to stick fanatically to them to lose weight, and that if they step out of line by as little as a biscuit they might as well give up. This is one reason why I do not agree with strict diets which dictate everything you can and cannot eat. Always remember, when discouraged, that you did not get fat overnight and you certainly will not get fat on one lapse.

★ **You do not need to count calories to lose weight effectively**. This is true, but being calorie-aware is important. Knowing where hidden fats are is the best way to control calorie intake.

★ **Fasting is the best way to lose weight.** Very sudden drops in calorie intake – or none at all, as in fasting – means that the body, aware that it is being starved, prepares for a famine. It starts to conserve energy by reducing the normal basal metabolic rate (BMR) and therefore cutting its normal calorific requirements. In addition, rather than burning fat from the bodily fat deposit stores that you so desperately want to lose, it starts consuming muscle tissue and carbohydrate stores as well. So this approach is flawed from the outset. When you start eating normally again, the body's first priority is to restock its depleted reserves for the next time you starve it. One of the first areas to be restocked are the depleted fat stores, which is why it is all too easy to end up where you started – a familiar scenario for most crash-dieters!
▷

Nine out of ten crash-dieters put all the weight back on within twelve months.

★ **No gain without pain.** You do not have to go hungry, starve yourself or suffer to lose weight. In fact, depriving yourself of food is the shortest route to failure. Keeping weight under control is a matter of matching daily calorie intake to daily calorie expenditure.For example, people who lead essentially sedentary lives, such as office workers, need fewer calories than someone who is physically active, such as a coal miner.

★ **Skipping breakfast is a diet.** People often think the best way to diet is to 'skip' breakfast and only have a mug of black coffee. But by the time we get up in the morning, we may not have eaten anything for up to twelve hours.

Breakfast kick-starts the metabolism and means we burn between 100 to 150 calories (equivalent of a slice of bread and butter) more than those who skip it! People who eat breakfast are also less likely to overeat at other times of the day, and more likely to avoid snacking and relying on calories from fat. There is some truth in the old adage: breakfast like a king, lunch like a prince, and dine like a pauper.

Going to work on an empty stomach also means our bodies will not be functioning at peak efficiency and mood, concentration and performance may be affected. So, go to work on an egg – or, better still, some porridge or muesli!

★ **Spot diets**. Many diets imply that you can target specific 'trouble' spots – usually thighs – when losing weight. In fact, spot-diets are a physiological impossibility. Our bodies lose fat from inside the abdominal cavity first, then from the face and between the shoulder blades, and then from the hips and thighs. Most people lose fat from places which are already quite slim – the main fat depots are the last to be lost.

This is probably the most common con trick that persists in the world of dieting, but belief in it continues and is demonstrated by the popularity of some of the biggest selling diet books and videos. Save your money!

★ **All fats are bad for you.** This is not true. For all their problems, fats are an essential part of our diet. The important thing is not to eat too many of them, and to select foods from the healthier polyunsaturated and mono-unsaturated fats group, instead of saturated (see page 16). ▷

It is important to concentrate on achieving a healthy diet and to be more active.

◁★ **Food-combination diets.** The idea behind food-combination diets, for example the Hay diet, is that we should not mix proteins and carbohydrates in the same meal, and should eat foods which restore the body's natural balance between acids and alkalis. What the idea fails to recognise is that almost all plant foods contain both protein and carbohydrate, for example rice, wheat, oats, maize and milk.

Of course, it is possible to lose weight by following a food combination diet, but, in my opinion, this has more to do with the type of foods advocated and their calorific content, rather than how they interact or 'combine' with each other!

★ **Grapefruit and pineapple diets.** The idea behind the grapefruit and pineapple diets is that they contain a 'magic' ingredient which, if you eat enough of it, means you can eat what you like of everything else. This is simply not true. Any weight loss is due to the change in the types of foods you eat.

★ **Lose 9 kg (20 lb) in two weeks.** It is a scientific impossibility to lose this much fat in two weeks. Most of the initial fast weight loss that we are so proud of achieving is actually not fat at all. It is due to water and carbohydrate loss. Sadly, burning off fat is a much slower process.

★ **Fast dieting improves your health.** This is the biggest con of all. Reaching your ideal weight range can, of course, have major health benefits, but getting there can actually damage health. The only healthy weight loss is a slow weight loss, the ideal figure being around 1 kg (2 lb) a week. Any more than this means you are very likely compromising your actual nutritional requirements.

The only healthy weight loss is a slow weight loss: around 1 kg (2 lb) a week.

Cellulite

This is the term coined by the health and beauty industry to describe the puckered orange-peel appearance of fat often found on women's thighs. Today women – even thin women – dread it. Aussie super model, Elle-the-body MacPherson, endeared herself to millions of British women when she admitted she had it; and the tabloids love showing their readers that the likes of Naomi Campbell and Pamela Anderson are not immune from it.

Cosmetic companies, beauty salons, slimming food manufacturers and plastic surgeons make millions preying on women's paranoia about cellulite. In reality, however, it is no different from any other type of fat. The sad and inevitable fact is that women have a greater tendency to store fat on their upper thighs and buttocks. This area is rich in connective-tissue fibres which form a mesh-like network rather like a string vest. When fat is deposited, it fills up the gaps giving a dimply appearance.

Why only women? Women's fat cells are substantially bigger and closer to the surface than men's, and the skin and tissue covering them is much thinner, making them more obvious. Age also does not favour women in this respect because, as we age, the connective tissue tends to weaken and break down, pushing the fat cells even closer to the surface.

Any suggestion that cellulite has anything to do with the accumulation of toxins in your body and that eliminating these from your diet (so-called anti-cellulite diets) can somehow get rid of them, is utter nonsense.

Likewise, anti-cellulite creams are, for the most part, a complete waste of time and money. There is some evidence that drugs, such as amino-phylline, can help to reduce cellulite but its inclusion in cosmetic products is of very dubious value.

Cellulite is just plain old fat and, like the fat in every other part of the body, can only be got rid of through a healthy programme of weight loss combined with exercise. Unfortunately, the hips and thighs are a natural fat storage area for many women and, with the best will in the world, are often the last store to be depleted.

Losing weight and toning up the muscles of the thigh and buttock will help improve the appearance of legs affected by cellulite, but I am afraid that there is no way of getting rid of it completely.

Very low-calorie diets: the biggest drawback of these diets is that they have an incredibly high failure rate. While they might be useful to help you look slimmer for your summer holiday, most are doomed to failure in the long term. Once you hit your target weight the chances are that you will return to your normal eating habits which were the reason you put on weight in the first place.

This is why most low calorie diet plans have only a five per cent chance of long-term success. Low calorie substitute foods, for example slimming drinks, make little sense to me. They do nothing to correct dietary problems and go against all the basic principles of successful long-term weight control. In fact, they can make matters worse by encouraging unhealthy and unnatural eating habits.

Severely restricted calorie intake only has a place in the treatment of severe obesity, under medical supervision.

WARNING

None of the medications mentioned in the following sections has any place in the management of weight control. They will cause temporary weight loss, but this is neither real nor sustainable nor any reason for using them. If you are offered any of them, refuse them. All of them can cause serious medical problems.

Slimming clinics: there are a growing number of private slimming clinics that promise rapid weight loss using a variety of pills and potions. These are undoubtedly popular with dieters because they offer a quick fix without all the hassle of healthy eating and exercise. Unfortunately they do not work, and are potentially dangerous.

Slimming pills containing diethylpropion and phenteramine can have any or all of the side-effects listed on the right (see Appetite suppressants opposite).

★ Addiction
★ Sleeplessness
★ Depression
★ Hallucinations
★ Palpitations
★ High blood pressure

Appetite suppressants: the use of these is at best highly controversial and at worst verging on malpractice. To quote the doctor's drug bible, the British National Formulary: 'Appetite suppressants are of no real value in the treatment of obesity since they do not improve the long-term outlook. Even worse the use of amphetamine-like drugs, diethylpropion (Tenuate Dospan) and phenteramine (Apisate), is not justified because any possible benefits are outweighed by the risks involved.'

In plain English, these drugs rarely, if ever, work in the long term, are potentially addictive and can cause serious physical and psychological side-effects.

The Department of Health is currently considering proposals to restrict the prescription of appetite suppressants. No legislation is in place as I write, but these proposals, and increasing medical anxieties about their use, have already led the manufacturers of Tenuate Dospan and Apisate to withdraw their products from the market.

My advice is to avoid slimming pills altogether. If you are offered them by a private clinic, refuse them, or at the very least consult your GP before taking any.

Thyroid hormone treatment: some people, desperate to lose weight, have even been offered thyroid hormone by unscrupulous slimming practitioners. This drug, available only on prescription, is for treating thyroid deficiency. It does cause weight loss by raising a person's basal metabolic rate (BMR), but it has no place in the treatment of healthy, albeit overweight people.

- ★ Palpitations
- ★ Life-threatening rhythm disturbances of the heart
- ★ Muscle cramps
- ★ Sweating
- ★ Diarrhoea
- ★ Dangerous weight loss

When taken by people with normal thyroid levels, thyroid hormone (thyroxine), can cause the listed symptoms.

Laxatives: other drug abuses include the use of laxatives. All they do is dramatically shorten the length of time that food spends travelling through the gut. While this may reduce the number of calories absorbed from food, it also reduces the amount of essential vitamins and minerals absorbed, and can lead to dangerous nutritional deficiencies. Long-term use can cause:

▶ Continual diarrhoea.
▶ Dehydration.
▶ Damage to both the lining and the muscles of the bowel wall.

Diuretics (water tablets): these reduce fluid retention by increasing our need to urinate. They also induce a state of mild dehydration and can create nutritional deficiencies through a loss of essential minerals. They should not be used without consulting your GP. Side-effects include:

▶ Low blood pressure.
▶ Gout.
▶ Severe skin rashes.
▶ Liver problems.
▶ Impotence.

Be more active

Remember, one of the chief reasons we are becoming a nation of fatties is that the majority of us are expending less energy – and using up fewer calories – on day-to-day activities. Despite our ever-growing waistlines, our average daily activity levels have fallen by a third over the past forty years. In calorific terms, this is a difference between using up about 2500 calories (a traffic warden) and 1800 calories (a secretary) a day.

None of this is surprising when you remember that, today, we use less energy on keeping warm, and sit in front of the television for an average of twenty-five to thirty hours a week. When we do go out, we use cars, lifts and escalators.

It is easy to see what a difference more exercise could make in our life. Consider, for example, the calorie needs of two women, one active, the other sedentary. The active one burns up about 2500 calories a day, the inactive about 1800. If both eat 2000 calories a day, the secretary will, in theory, put on weight at the rate of about 1 kg (2 lb) a month and the traffic warden will lose around 1.5 kg (3 lb) a month. So, let's just accept that no weight-loss programme can be complete – really successful – without combining it with exercise (for exercise details, see Chapter Two).

HAVE FUN, LOSE WEIGHT!

SUCCESSFUL DIETING

The only way to control your weight in the long term is to take a long hard look at your eating habits and try to change them for the better over a period of months. No one is asking you to become a health-food fanatic, but any steps you take towards healthier eating (see the food section of this chapter) will be accompanied by better weight control and a general improvement in well-being. For a successful diet plan follow these basic guidelines:

★ Have realistic expectations. Go for an achievable and sustainable weight loss that puts you at the higher level of your ideal weight range (see chart on page 44). Aim for a loss of 1 kg (2 lb) a week. Don't worry if you are a little bit over your ideal weight. It may take you a while to hit your target weight, but, once you do, you are far more likely to stay there.

★ Take a long hard look at the food you are eating and see if you can identify the problem areas. The two main culprits are too much fat and sugar. Use low-fat alternatives such as skimmed milk, low-fat yoghurts and cheese whenever possible.

★ Prepare foods in such a way that you keep fat content to a minimum, for example, grill, bake or steam instead of frying.

★ Remove the skin and fat from meat products.

★ Avoid all types of confectionery.

★ Try not to add sugar to drinks and foodstuffs.

★Increase fibre in your diet (see page 24). High-fibre food tends to be low in calories and high in vitamins and minerals. It also helps the bowel to work at peak efficiency.

★ Do not skip breakfast and eat regular meals throughout the day.

★ Avoid snacking – if you must eat between meals, then eat fresh fruit or raw vegetables.

★ Combine healthy eating with a more active lifestyle.

★Only weigh yourself once a week – day-to-day variations of 1–1.5 kg (2–3 lb) either way are normal fluctuations.

★ Healthy weight loss is slow – about 1 kg (2 lb) a week.
★ Crash diets invariably fail – and can be dangerous.
★ Successful dieting is always combined with an increase in physical activity – exercise.
★ Avoid slimming aids, such as pills and laxatives. They all have potentially dangerous side-effects.

Closing thoughts

Food is one of life's great pleasures, and it is surprisingly easy to make our diet healthier. If we follow the few basic guidelines in this chapter, we can be sure that any progress we make is a step in the right direction. There is not so very much to remember and you will certainly find that when you achieve one goal, the others will naturally follow on. For example, a high-fibre diet tends also to be high in fresh produce and low in fat; a low-fat diet is higher in fibre and fresh produce. A healthy diet really can be happy eating.

The Department of Health emphasise the need to encourage children to eat more vegetables and fruit.

Fourteen-day healthy-eating meal plan guide

★ Eat at least five portions of fruit and vegetables a day.
★ Reduce total fat intake, particularly saturated fat.
★ Increase fibre intake.
★ Reduce sugar and salt intake.
★ Aim to get half your daily calories from carbohydrates found in starchy foods, such as bread, potatoes, rice, pasta and breakfast cereals.

This fourteen-day healthy-eating meal plan , which includes ideas for packed lunches, sandwich fillings and healthy snacks, has been designed to get us off to a good start and show us just how easy and enjoyable it can be to eat a healthy diet. It is suitable for the whole family – women, men and children. People with large appetites simply need to eat bigger portions of the breakfast, lunch and evening meal suggestions, or enjoy more of the healthy snack suggestions. The evening meals are more substantial than the lunches but you can adapt the meal plan to suit your lifestyle.

Fruit and vegetables: aim for five or more servings from this group each day. One serving is equivalent to:

▶ 2–3 tablespoons root or green vegetables, cooked or raw
▶ 1 small salad
▶ 1 piece fresh fruit
▶ 2 tablespoons canned fruit
▶ 3 dried apricots
▶ 1 small glass fruit juice

We should aim to eat at least five servings of fruit and/or vegetables a day. This may sound like a difficult target to achieve, but if you spread the servings throughout the day you will find it is easier than you think. Try to have at least one serving of fruit and vegetables at each meal, and a couple of pieces of fruit as snacks throughout the day. It really does not matter if these are fresh, frozen, canned or dried.

Fruit and vegetables are low in fat and calories. They contain dietary fibre – particularly soluble fibre – which can help to reduce high blood cholesterol levels and provide antioxidants, such as beta-carotene and vitamin C, which help to protect the body from the damaging effects of free radicals believed to cause cancer and coronary heart disease. Leafy green vegetables, such as spinach and broccoli, provide the B vitamin folic acid, an important vitamin for women of child-bearing age.

Bread, grains, rice, breakfast cereals, pasta, potatoes: aim for between 5–11 servings from this group each day. One serving is equivalent to:

▶ 3 tablespoons breakfast cereal
▶ 2 tablespoons porridge oats or muesli
▶ 1 slice of bread or 1 bread roll
▶ 1 scone, muffin or teacake
▶ 1 egg-sized potato or 3 small new potatoes
▶ 1 tablespoon cooked rice or pasta
▶ 3 crispbreads or 2 cream crackers
▶ 1 digestive biscuit

Foods from this group provide fibre, protein, vitamins and minerals. These are the foods to fill up on – and should provide most of our calories. Many people worry that these foods are fattening, but eaten, in fact, by themselves they are low in fat. It is, of course, important to remember that if they are combined with large amounts of fat they are high in calories. For example, a slice of wholemeal bread contains about seventy-five calories, but this is easily doubled by spreading a generous amount of butter on the bread.

Dairy products: (milk, cheese, yoghurt, fromage frais) – aim for between 2–3 servings from this group each day. The amounts for one serving are listed. Dairy products provide many useful nutrients, particularly calcium, which is important for strong bones. They also contain large amounts of fat, a high proportion of which is saturated. For this reason, they should be eaten in moderation. Using reduced-fat varieties can help to control fat intake.

▶ 200 ml (7 fl oz) milk.
▶ small piece of cheese, the size of a match box (40 g/1½ oz).
▶ small tub of cottage cheese.
▶ 1 small pot yoghurt or fromage frais (150 g/5 oz).

Meat, poultry, fish, eggs, nuts and pulses(beans and lentils):
aim for 2–3 servings from this group a day. One serving is equivalent to:

▶ 50–75 g (2–3 oz) lean meat, chicken, offal or oily fish
▶ 125–150 g (4–5 oz) white fish

▶ 1 egg
▶ 3 tablespoons cooked beans or pulses or peas
▶ 2 tablespoons nuts, peanut butter

Foods from this group provide protein, fat, vitamins and minerals. Like dairy products, they can also contain lots of fat so they need to be eaten in moderation. Choose lean meat and trim off any fat before cooking. Fish is quick to cook, versatile and extremely nutritious: health experts suggest that we should try to eat fish at least twice a week. White fish, such as cod and haddock, are very low in fat. Oily fish such as sardines, pilchards, herrings, fresh (not canned) tuna and salmon, contain more fat but of the kind known as Omega-3, which nutritionists believe is helpful in preventing heart disease (see Benefits of fish, page 24).

Fatty and sugary foods: although a small amount of fat is essential in our diet, most of us eat far too much (see Fats, page 13). Diets that contain high levels of saturated fat are known to increase the risk of heart disease and certain types of cancer. For good health we need a balance between the three different types of fat:

▶ Monounsaturated fat – found in olive oil, peanuts, avocado pears and rapeseed oil.
▶ Polyunsaturated fat – found mainly in vegetable and seed oils, oily fish and lean meat.
▶ Saturated fats – found mainly in animal fats such as the fat in meat and dairy products.

The most important thing to remember is that whatever type of fat you choose – use it sparingly.

Like fat, most of us eat far more sugar than is recommended for good health. While it is not necessary to avoid sugar altogether, it makes good sense to think about the amount of sugar we eat. It provides 'empty calories' which most of us could do without.

Packed lunches: food left for long periods of time in a warm place provides the ideal conditions for the growth of bacteria which cause food poisoning. A packed lunch, therefore, should always be kept in an insulated cool bag. Even in winter months this is important, because satchels and school bags are left in warm classrooms or cloakrooms.

▶ Lentil soup/vegetable soup with wholemeal roll or cheese scone
  Low-fat fruit yoghurt
  Small carton of fruit juice
  Banana

▶ Chicken pitta pockets
  Carrot sticks
  Packet of reduced-fat crisps
  Small bunch of grapes
  Small carton of fruit juice

▶ Sardine salad finger roll
  A few cherry tomatoes
  Apple
  Small carton of fruit juice

Sandwich fillings: suggestions

Meat fillings
Wafer-thin ham, reduced-fat cream cheese and grated carrot
Smoked turkey, avocado pear and alfalfa sprouts
Salmon and cucumber
Chicken salad and coleslaw
Tuna and sweetcorn (use tuna in brine or water and mix with a little reduced-fat mayonnaise and some canned sweetcorn)
Smoked salmon and reduced-fat cream cheese
Chicken tikka with yoghurt and mint dressing and mango chutney
Smoked ham and mustard

Vegetarian fillings
Edam cheese and tomato relish
Brie and black grape

Egg and cress
Reduced-fat soft cheese and apricots
Stilton and pear
Reduced-fat cottage cheese and marmite
Reduced-fat cream cheese and pineapple
Roasted red pepper and reduced-fat cream cheese

Vegan fillings
Peanut butter and cucumber
Hummus and grated carrot
Peanut butter and jam
Banana (mash the banana with a little lemon juice, add cinnamon to taste)
Roasted vegetables (e.g. peppers and courgettes)
Hummus and alfafa
Peanut butter and apple

Did you know?
The vitamins in fruit and vegetables can be easily destroyed during storage, preparation and cooking. To get the most from your fruit and vegetables:

★ Buy 'little and often' rather than in huge quantities.
★ Store vegetables in a cool dark place, ideally for no more than three days.
★ Cut vegetables into large chunks so less surface area is exposed (vitamin C is lost when cut surfaces come into contact with the air).
★ Never leave vegetables standing in water before cooking.
★ Microwave cooking, steaming or stir-frying are the best methods to use for cooking vegetables. Boiling vegetables in large quantities of water can remove up to seventy per cent of the vitamin C. If you do boil vegetables, use the minimum amount of water and add the vegetables only when it is boiling. Once the vegetables are cooked use the water that remains to make gravy, sauce, soup or stock.
★ Eat food as soon as you can after it is prepared. Keeping food warm results in more vitamins being lost.

MEAL PLAN: Week 1

	MONDAY	TUESDAY	WEDNESDAY
BREAKFASTS ★ A bowl of high-fibre breakfast cereal can provide as much as half of the recommended daily amount of dietary fibre.	Fruit juice Wholegrain cereal with semi-skimmed milk and a chopped banana Wholemeal toast, thin scrape of butter or margarine and reduced-sugar jam or mamalade, yeast extract or honey	Fruit juice Poached egg on whole-meal toast ★ Breakfast is particularly important when you are watching your weight. Skipping breakfast simply means that you are more likely to get hungry and start to nibble around mid-morning.	Fruit juice Fruity porridge
LUNCHES	Sardine salad Granary bread roll with thin scrape of butter or margarine Apple or another piece of fresh fruit	Lentil soup French bread 1 orange or 2 satsumas Did you know? ★ Canned fruit in syrup has twice as much sugar as fresh fruit. Use fruit canned in natural juice or water.	Mushroom omelette Grilled tomato Wholemeal fruit scone or muffin Low-fat fruit yoghurt
EVENING MEALS	Jacket potato with chilli con carne and sweetcorn Fruit yoghurt	Vegetable lasagne Green salad Baked fruit salad	Tandoori chicken Vegetable curry Boiled rice Melon and kiwi salad

Did you know?
★ Wholemeal flour contains more fibre and B vitamins than white. If you would like to use wholemeal flour but find it a little heavy, start by using half wholemeal and half white, and then gradually increase the proportion of wholemeal and reduce the white.

THURSDAY	FRIDAY	SATURDAY	SUNDAY
Fruit juice Branflakes, with a few dried apricots and semi-skimmed milk Wholemeal toast, thin scrape butter or margarine and reduced-sugar jam or marmalade, yeast extract, or honey	Fruit juice Apple muesli (soak some muesli in semi-skimmed milk overnight in the fridge and, just before serving, add a grated apple and a spoonful of yoghurt)	Fruit juice Fruit compôte with yoghurt Wholemeal toast ★ Despite the fact that many nutritionists consider breakfast the most important meal of the day, nearly half of us choose to start the day without it.	Fruit juice Orange and grapefruit segments Scrambled eggs on toast
Ham salad sandwich Low-fat fruit yoghurt	Chicken pitta pockets (place a wholemeal pitta under a hot grill for a few minutes to warm, then add some strips of cooked chicken breast, coleslaw and shredded lettuce) Fresh fruit salad or pine-apple canned in natural juice	Vegetable soup with garlic croûtons Smoked mackerel pâté with granary baguette Cherry tomato and celery salad Banana and custard	Roast chicken Roast potatoes Roast parsnips Braised red cabbage Apple and apricot crumble
Macaroni and leeks in cheese sauce with a breadcrumb topping Mixed salad Frozen yoghurt with baked banana	Fisherman's pie French beans and courgettes Baked apples with a date and walnut filling, served with a little Greek yoghurt	Stir-fried pork with noodles Vanilla ice-cream with peach sauce (to make the peach sauce, drain the juice from a can of peaches, liquidise until smooth, adding a little juice if necessary)	Wholemeal Quiche Lorraine Pasta salad Carrot and nut salad Fresh fruit salad

★ Breakfast like a king, lunch like a prince, and dine like a pauper. However, if your lifestyle makes this impossible, try it out, say, on a Sunday. You'll feel better. Especially if you also take some exercise.

	MONDAY	TUESDAY	WEDNESDAY	
BREAKFASTS	Fruit juice Wholegrain cereal, semi-skimmed milk, chopped banana. Wholemeal toast, thin scrape butter or margarine and reduced-sugar jam or mamalade, yeast extract, or honey	Fruit juice Scrambled eggs on toast **Did you know?** ★Fruit and vegetables contain dietary fibre – particularly soluble fibre – which can help to reduce high blood cholesterol levels and provide antioxidants.	Fruit juice Fruity porridge	
LUNCHES	Baked beans on whole-meal toast Fruit salad	Cheese and tomatoes on toast (thinly slice one large beefsteak tomato, place on a slice of wholemeal toast, sprinkle with a little oregano, top with grated cheese and place under a hot grill until the cheese has melted) Fruit yoghurt	Pilchard salad sandwich Packet of reduced-fat crisps Small bunch of grapes	
EVENING MEALS	Shepherd's pie (add some frozen peas and sweetcorn to the mince and make the topping from a mixture of mashed potato and celeriac, cooking the celeriac in the same way as the potato) Orange and mango jelly	Tomato soup Ham and pineapple pizza Mixed salad Fruit kebabs **HEALTHY-EATING TIP** ★ Persuading children to eat vegetables is not always easy. Concentrate on those vegetables that your child will eat, introducing others in such dishes as spaghetti bolognese and shepherd's pie. Add just a little at first and then gradually increase the amount.	Pork and pepper kebabs Tzatziki (yoghurt and cucumber dip) Boiled rice Dried fruit compôte with frozen yoghurt	

THURSDAY	FRIDAY	SATURDAY	SUNDAY
Fruit juice Wholegrain cereal, semi-skimmed milk, with a few chopped apricots Wholemeal toast, thin scrape butter or margarine and reduced-sugar jam or marmalade, or yeast extract, or honey	Fruit juice Apple muesli (see Friday, Week 1)	Fruit juice Pancakes served with fruit compôte and yoghurt Wholemeal toast	Fruit juice Grilled bacon, scrambled egg, grilled mushrooms and tomatoes Wholemeal toast

SNACKS

Apricot smoothie . Ready-to-eat dried apricots. Breakfast cereals. Fresh fruit. Flapjack. Mixed nuts and raisins. Banana sandwich. Wholemeal muffin or scone. Oat cakes. Digestive biscuits.

THURSDAY	FRIDAY	SATURDAY	SUNDAY
Jacket potato with ratatouille topped with a little grated cheese Flapjack	Scrambled eggs on wholemeal toast Fruit yoghurt	Carrot and coriander soup Bagel with reduced-fat cream cheese and smoked salmon Fresh fruit salad	Poached salmon New potatoes Ratatouille and green beans Apple strudel with a little Greek yoghurt

Did you know?

★ Frozen vegetables contain just as much, in fact sometimes more, vitamin C than fresh.

★ To make the best use of the fibre and vitamins in fruit and vegetables, which are stored in or just under the skin, wash thoroughly and eat them with the skin on.

THURSDAY	FRIDAY	SATURDAY	SUNDAY
Baked cod steaks with a rich tomato sauce Reduced-fat oven chips Broccoli and carrots Fruit salad	Spaghetti bolognese Poached pears with chocolate sauce	Chicken casserole with mashed potato Spinach and mangetout Bread and butter pudding	Hummus with sticks of raw vegetables (carrot, celery, strips of red and yellow pepper, cucumber) Reduced-fat pâté French bread Vanilla ice-cream with strawberry sauce (to make the sauce, drain the juice from a can of strawberries in natural juice, liquidise until smooth, adding a little juice if necessary. Use fresh strawberries when they are in season)

Did you know?

★ Oil-rich fish, such as salmon, herring, trout and mackerel, are rich in Omega-3 fatty acids, a type of polyunsaturated fat which can help protect against coronary heart disease and strokes by making blood less 'sticky' and therefore less likely to clot. Nutritionists recommend us to eat at least two fish-based meals each week.

✉ Useful addresses

▶ British Diabetic Association, 10 Queen Anne Street, London W1M 0BD. Telephone: 0171 323 1531.

▶ British Heart Foundation, 14 Fitzhardinge Street, London W1H 4DH. Telephone: 0171 935 0185.

▶ British Nutrition Foundation, The, High Holborn House, 52–4 High Holborn, London WC1V 6RQ. Telephone: 0171 404 6504. Leaflets and information available.

▶ Diet Breakers, Barford St Michael, Banbury, Oxford OX15 0UA. Telephone: 01869 337070. Help for those who want to break free from the diet–binge cycle. Produce booklet (send sae) and run workshops.

▶ Eating Disorders Association, Sackville Place, 44–8 Magdalen Street, Norwich NR3 1JU. Telephone: 01603 621414.

▶ Fish Foundation, The, PO Box 24, Tiverton, Devon EX16 4QQ. Telephone: 01884 257547.

▶ Health Education Authority, The, Customer Services Department, Marston Book Services Ltd, PO Box 269, Abingdon, Oxon OX14 4GN. Telephone: 0171 404 6504. Produce leaflets on wide range of health subjects, including healthy eating, exercise and alcohol.

▶ Hyperactive Children's Support Group, 71 Whyke Lane, Chichester, W. Sussex PO19 2LD. Telephone: 01903 725182.

▶ Imperial Cancer Research Fund, PO Box 123, Lincoln's Inn Fields, London WC2A 3PX. Telephone: 0171 242 0200.

▶ Meat and Livestock Commission, PO Box 44, Winterhill House, Snowden Drive, Milton Keynes MK6 1AX. Telephone: 01908 677577.

▶ Ministry of Agriculture, Fisheries and Food, The, Helpline, Room 11, Whitehall Place West, London SW1A 2HH. Telephone: 01645 335577. Leaflets available with information on, for example, a healthy diet, food safety and understanding food labels.

▶ National Dairy Council, 5–7 John Princes Street, London W1M 0AP. Telephone: 0171 499 7822.

▶ Vegetarian Society (UK), The, Parkdale, Dunham Road, Altrincham, Cheshire WA14 4QG. Telephone: 01619 280793. Produce information pack and run residential cookery courses.

CHAPTER TWO

'EXERCISE IS BORING AND IT HURTS – NOT!'

★ Just a small increase in activity will bring about health improvements.

★ The less you do at the moment, the more you will benefit from activity.

★ The concept of 'no pain no gain' has no place in any exercise programme.

★ Walking, housework, gardening, playing with the children all count.

★ If you do join a gym, seek qualified advice and help before embarking on any fitness programme.

SUNDAY'S CHOICE

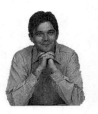

Get Fit

Exercise seems to have been hijacked by the body beautiful brigade and become more about looking good than improving our health. Gyms have become the ultimate places to show off that perfect body (if you are lucky) rather than a place to develop a healthy one.

Of course, getting rid of some excess weight and improving the way we look is a very powerful motivation to exercise for some of us, but it is wrong to think that to get healthy we need to aim at looking like someone from the set of *Baywatch*.

Likewise, the misconception that to reap any health benefits we have to engage in vigorous, fanatical, continuous exercise is probably why so many people remain inactive – seven out of ten men and eight out of ten women in the UK do not do enough physical activity to get any health benefit.

A lack of activity increases our risk of coronary heart disease.

So, if the word exercise puts you off by conjuring up grim images of overzealous, overmuscled and over-tanned aerobic teachers you have my deepest sympathies. Now that my rugby days are over I, too, have no desire to don the male equivalent of the leotard and trot off to the gym three times a week.

The good news, however, is that we don't have to. There is now growing support for, and interest in, the benefits of increasing our day-to-day levels of activity, rather than taking up a specific form of exercise.

Our modern lifestyle has a lot to answer for. For example, the average person in England now watches over twenty-six hours of television a week compared with thirteen hours in the 1960s. Excessive television viewing – and we do not even need to get out of our chair to change channels – has been identified as one of the major causes of inactivity and childhood and adolescent obesity. Likewise, on the work front, only one in five men and one in ten women are now employed in physically active occupations. In addition, cars, lifts, escalators, sedentary jobs mean we do far less than we were designed to do.

Just think back to how we evolved. Humans are designed to be hunter-gatherers. One of the few races that followed this lifestyle this century were the aborigines in the outback of Australia. At that time, a typical day for them entailed a five- to ten-mile brisk walk, collecting foodstuffs and hunting as they went. They did not run marathons or pump iron, and yet they were in peak physical condition, their bodies shaped by evolutionary pressures to be perfect for their lifestyle. Our lifestyles in the so-called developed world, however, have changed beyond all recognition in the last hundred years, and it will take our bodies thousands of evolutionary years to make the equivalent adjustment.

So, what this means is that you don't have to turn up at your local health club for three hours a week. In fact nothing could be furtherfrom the truth.

What we should be trying to achieve is an increase of activity in our basic day-to-day activities. This approach where the emphasis is on increasing overall activity level rather than trotting down to the gym is now getting more recognition.

The other advantage about this approach is that it leads to a permanent change in activity levels – it works on the same principle as changing an unhealthy diet to a healthy diet. A six-week or even a year's sudden and temporary interest in the gym is not going to be of any lasting benefit, but persevering and changing our basic activity level permanently will be.

So, this chapter is not about developing a beautiful body or training to run a marathon, it's about a permanent change in lifestyle that improves our health.

Health benefits of activity

Perhaps the best way to emphasise the health benefits of exercise, whatever form it takes, or increase in physical activity, is to look at the health risks of inactivity. For example, in America it has been estimated that as many as one in ten deaths are caused by a lack of exercise. This adds up to 250 000 people every year.

A lack of activity increases our risk of coronary heart disease (see Rates of coronary heart disease, page 13) by as much as two and a half times – putting it right up there in terms of a health hazard with smoking and high blood pressure.

But it is not just our hearts which benefit from exercise – every part of our body can get healthier. It is impossible to put a stronger case for any health benefit (apart from giving up smoking). Here is a quick guide to the good you will be doing yourself with more activity:

Heart and lungs: like any other muscle, the heart becomes stronger with use which means that even everyday activities put less stress on it. Regular exercise also improves the ability of the heart and lungs to supply essential nutrients and oxygen to all parts of the body and remove unwanted by-products.

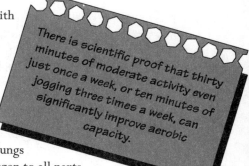

There is scientific proof that thirty minutes of moderate activity even just once a week, or ten minutes of jogging three times a week, can significantly improve aerobic capacity.

Cholesterol: regular exercise increases the level of HDL cholesterol (the good form) and reduces our chances of fatty plaques developing in our arteries.

Blood pressure: exercise can reduce the blood pressure of people with mild hypertension, and also dampens the inevitable rise of blood pressure found in middle age in Western society.

Bones: bone is a living tissue and its density increases until the mid-thirties and then starts to drop off slightly. In women, the decrease is particularly dramatic after the menopause. If bone density drops below a certain threshold level, the risk of bone fractures increases. Many factors affect bone density, but exercise – particularly weight-bearing exercise – is crucial. Regular use of joints and muscles also helps them remain supple.

Back pain: one of the commonest causes of back pain is a sedentary lifestyle. People who do not exercise have weaker back muscles and increase their risk of injury. It is estimated that eight out of ten people in the Western world suffer back pain at some time or other, and in the UK it results in 11.5 million lost working days a year.

Weight loss: exercise helps us to burn up calories that would otherwise be converted to fat. It also increases body muscle which increases our resting metabolic rate.

Diabetes: diabetics do not produce any, or enough, insulin which is the hormone we need to control the uptake of sugar in the blood by cells. Although some people develop diabetes early in life, most develop it in middle-age (non-insulin dependent diabetes, NIDD). Doctors now believe that exercise and good nutrition can prevent many cases of NIDD.

Mood and self-esteem: exercise increases the levels of brain chemicals called endorphins – and it is these which are responsible for the euphoric high feeling after exercise. Many studies report less stress, irritation, depression and anxiety after exercise. And, in addition to improving mood disorders, endorphins can relieve bodily aches and pains. Exercise, in fact, is a great and natural way of relieving mental and physical stress.

The bare minimum

The most widely quoted recommendation for the amount of exercise we should all be doing, and the one endorsed by the Sports Council, is twenty to sixty minutes of moderate to high intensity endurance exercise performed at least three times a week.

That's all very well, but it is by no means a popular option. And the problem I see with it is that it carries an inherent implication that if we do anything less, we are wasting our time. In truth, this is not the case.

Lower levels of activity can still result in health improvements. The greatest benefits from any increase in activity occur when the true couch potato starts to become just a little active. Thereafter, the improvements become less for a similar increase in activity. In other words, there is more benefit from going from a couch potato to slightly active than when someone of already moderate activity really gets physical. There is scientific proof that thirty minutes of moderate activity even just once a week, or ten minutes of jogging three times a week, can significantly improve aerobic capacity and body composition in previously sedentary people.

But even this ignores the distinction between exercising to get fit and exercising to get healthy. What if you do not want to get fit, but you want to do a little to reduce your chances of a heart attack,

Remember that all increases in activity should be gradual.

or diabetes or hypertension, or one of the other chronic degenerative diseases linked with inactivity? In other words, strange as it may seem, you want to improve your health.

I don't know about you, but I don't need or want to be able to run ten miles a day but I do want to keep healthy. Long-term studies show that the type of physical activity associated with good health are activities such as walking, stair-climbing, gardening and household chores, rather than activities such as jogging, cycling or tennis, which can produce a multitude of sports injuries. In other words there has been a U-turn on the idea that we need to perform a bout of continuous exercise for twenty minutes or longer to achieve health benefits. Instead, a whole series of short bouts of activity spread throughout the day will do the job just as well, if not better. Recently the American College of Sports Medicine produced some official recommendations endorsing this view. It advises that everyone should tot up thirty minutes or more of moderate intensity physical activity on most, or all, days of the week.

If we do this all at once, it is the equivalent of walking 3 km (2 miles) a day at a brisk pace, but we don't have to set aside thirty minutes during the day — we just need to be more active throughout it. For example, walking up the stairs instead of taking the lift or escalator, walking short distances instead of driving count, as do gardening, housework, dancing or playing with the kids — as long as all these activities are carried out at an intensity correlating with brisk walking.

Scottish doctors showed how easy it is to encourage a general day-to-day increase in physical activity. According to a study published in the British Medical Journal, they placed signs saying Stay Healthy, Save Time, Use the Stairs on a city-centre underground station, where both the stairs and escalators (two sets of fifteen steps) were side by side. Before the signs were introduced, under one in eight men and one in twenty women used the stairs rather than the escalator. Once the signs were in place, these figures increased to more than one in five men and one in eight women. Not surprisingly the Health Education Board for Scotland is now employing this strategy.

Having said all this, remember that all increases in activity should be gradual. If you have long been sedentary, then start off with just a few minutes, gradually working up to longer time spans. I am not denying anywhere in this chapter that the more you do, the more you will benefit, but I would rather see people start off slowly increasing their levels of physical activity rather than go for it with an overenthusiasm that could then put them off at the beginning.

The most important thing about this recommendation for a steady increase in activity is that it is realistic. I can fit it into my life and most of my patients could, too. More to the point, all the excuses against exercising, such as 'I'm too busy,' 'I'm not sporty,' 'I'm unfit,' 'I'm too tired,' 'I'm too fat,' fall by the wayside.

So, take heart, an active lifestyle does not require a regimented vigorous exercise programme. Small changes that increase daily physical activity will enable individuals to reduce their risk of chronic disease and will contribute to an enhanced quality of life.

What about the children?

Much is being written in the press about the generation of couch potatoes we are now raising. However a distinction has to be made between our children's fitness and activity levels. According to research carried out at the Children's Health and Research Centre at the University of Exeter, our children today are as fit as children of other countries and are no less fit than their grandparents were at the same age. Our downfall is without doubt their activity levels.

The Exeter researchers examined this aspect in over 700 ten- to sixteen-year-olds and discovered that forty-seven per cent of girls and thirty-eight per cent of boys did not experience the equivalent of a ten-minute brisk walk during the three days they were monitored. In primary schoolchildren, the figures were twenty-eight per cent for girls and twenty-one per cent for boys.

This lack of activity is giving rise to great concern, particularly for the health of girls, as inactive children tend to grow up as inactive adults. So, although this lack of activity is not affecting children's fitness during childhood, it will certainly affect their fitness when they become adults. The saying 'Old habits die hard' is certainly true, so the more children do now, the more likely they are to be active later in life.

Although lounging around watching television and videos, and playing computer games, is largely blamed for children's lack of physical activity, the experts believe that other factors, such as being driven to and from school, may be even more important. For example, four times as many children are now driven to and from school than twenty years ago. Doubtless much of this has come about because of parents' concern for their children's safety in traffic-dominated areas, but some efforts need to be made if we are to balance these factors and, for our children's sake, improve their activity levels.

There are also major differences to be considered between how we raise boys and girls. For example, thirty per cent of boys are allowed to use their bikes after dark compared with just ten per cent of girls. The reason for this is obvious, but sexism is also at play in another way – exercise and sport are still stereotyped as masculine pursuits.

There has been a lot of interest recently in the role that physical education plays in the National Curriculum and Prime Minister John Major has said that two hours a week should be spent on sport and physical exercise. In reality, at the moment, less than half of our schoolchildren are achieving this. The Prime Minister is also very keen on team and competitive sports, but, likewise in reality, there is very little evidence that this is being put into effect.

One problem, from the girls' point of view, may be that team games tend to alienate them and they seem to prefer individual physical activities. Maybe things will improve more quickly if more effort is put into encouraging the types of exercise and physical activities that appeal to them, especially those activities that can be continued into adult life. After all, finding the time to exercise can be difficult enough in adult life without adding the complication of organising other people's busy schedules so that a game of netball, for example, can get off the ground. Whatever the approach, for girls and for boys, all the efforts will be richly rewarded if we can change our couch potato generation into more active people for the benefit of their adult life.

What about the elderly?

Exercise is particularly important for the elderly. Even healthy older people can lose physical strength at one to two per cent a year and power at three to four per cent – a decline which occurs even more dramatically if they experience an illness or undergo surgery. The resulting weakness can have dramatic consequences on their day-to-day life and activities. Women are

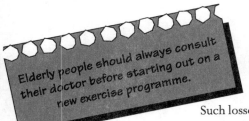

Elderly people should always consult their doctor before starting out on a new exercise programme.

particularly vulnerable to such losses because they have less muscle strength to lose in the first place. Such losses can make all the difference to being able to get in and out of the bath and climbing stairs.

Strength is the measure of force that a person can exert; power reflects the speed at which this strength can be exerted. On a day-to-day basis, the loss of power is probably more important. For example, it is power rather than strength that prevents a sudden loss of balance or a stumble turning into a fall.

Research at the Royal Free Hospital, London, revealed that women aged between seventy-five and ninety-three years who trained three times a week, for twenty minutes, for twelve weeks, increased their strength by as much as twenty-four to thirty per cent – equivalent to a person sixteen to twenty years younger. So, who says we cannot turn the clock back.

This training involved strength increasing exercises which could be done easily at home. After warming-up exercises – always essential before starting an exercise session – (see Warm up, cool down, page 78) the women were taught a series of exercises ranging from simple leg-lifts, while seated, to arm exercises which entailed lifting 750 g (1 ½ lb) bags of rice. Full details of this exercise programme are available in booklet form from Research Into Ageing, the charity which funded the work (see Useful addresses on page 84).

If you prefer to join a group, rather than exercise at home, your local council will have a list of all over-fifties and senior citizens' classes.

Before starting any exercise programme, it is important to consult your doctor. While exercise benefits everyone, certain forms are not wise for some people.

How much, how often?

Obviously the Sports Council recommendation of twenty to sixty minutes of moderate- to high-intensity endurance exercise, three times a week, is a good level to aim for – although bear in mind what I said above, that less is not a waste of time.

The most important benefit of a training programme is aerobic fitness

MAKING THE MOST OF A GYM

The bare minimum is one thing, but if you are keen to take on a bit more then great! More intense and formal types of exercise can reap major benefits.

But be warned, one of the commonest problems doctors meet in general practice is injured patients who, having taken up a formal exercise programme, are now physically hurt in one way or another, disillusioned, and giving up after only six weeks. Our surgeries, for example, in the middle of February, are full of people who have embarked on their new-found quest for fitness as a result of a hastily thought out New Year's resolution!

I cannot stress enough the importance of having realistic expectations about what you can and cannot achieve, and the importance of seeking expert advice before starting.

Being taught how to warm up (see Warm up, cool down, page 78), how to stretch, and what exercises to do to achieve your goals not only reduces the chance of injury but makes it far more likely that you will achieve what you set out to do. This, in turn, makes it more likely that you will continue and derive long-term health benefits.

(see What is aerobic exercise? below). The heart is the most vital muscle in the body and all exercise programmes should be aimed at getting it into shape before you work on the rest of your body.

Achieving the right intensity is a source of great confusion. A good rule of thumb that you are not overdoing it, is that you should be able to talk easily during aerobic exercise. If you can't, you are probably pushing yourself too hard. If you follow a measured approach, you should notice a marked improvement in your fitness level within four to six weeks, and, instead of sitting in your doctor's surgery nursing a torn muscle, you will be enjoying a new lease of life.

What is aerobic exercise?

Any type of exercise that uses the large muscle groups of the body, raises the heart rate, makes you sweat, increases breathing rate and can be sustained for more than a few minutes can be regarded as aerobic.

Some people seem to believe that just their presence in the gym is sufficient to get fit, even though they may be exerting themselves less than they would if they were running upstairs at home or carrying out some other ordinary task.

Getting your heart into shape is surprisingly easy if you follow a few basic rules. Top athletes have been using science to optimise their training for years and the same basic principles apply to anyone embarking on a new fitness programme.

All that you need to do is exercise hard enough to raise your pulse rate into what is known as the Cardiac Training Range (CTR). Doing any less is unlikely to give you any cumulative training benefit, and pushing yourself harder is actually a waste of time and effort. All you need to do is measure your heart rate and do a bit of simple maths. The easiest way to work out your heart rate is to take your pulse during a workout. First, find your pulse on your neck or wrist. Count the number of beats in twenty seconds and multiply this by three to get the beats per minute. This can be easier said than done when you are on a rowing machine. A more accurate way, which definitely saves a lot of hassle if you can afford it, is to use a heart rate monitor. These are available from most good sports shops and gyms, and cost from £70 upwards.

The CTR is the same for men and women, and you can work out your own CTR by using the following formula:

The figure 220, minus your age, gives you your maximum heart rate and this figure should never be exceeded. The CTR is sixty-five to eighty-five per cent of this figure.
Let me give you an example for a thirty-five year old.
220-35 = 185; 65 per cent of 185 is 120; 85 per cent of 185 is 157
Making the CTR 120–157.

Don't be put off by the maths, any self-respecting gym will have a chart on the wall showing what your particular CTR is.

All you need to do is creep into the bottom part of this range for twenty minutes, preferably three times a week. This does not include your warm-up and cool-down periods – both of which are essential to prevent injury (see Warm up, cool down, below). What this basically means is that you can minimise and optimise your physical effort. When you first start, a brisk walk will probably put you into your CTR. But as you get fitter and fitter, you will have to push harder and harder.

WARM UP, COOL DOWN

Overtight muscles can lead to poor posture, and tense painful necks and backs. Unfortunately, as we get older, we all become less supple and flexible. We can, however, slow down this process by practising simple muscle-stretching exercises (see A good stretch, opposite). It is a good idea to do these three to seven times a week, even if you are not taking part in an exercise programme.

Warming up: cold tense muscles are prone to injury which is why you should never jump on to your exercise bike or stepping or rowing machine without doing some simple stretches. The following points should also be kept in mind:

★ Never use the body's momentum to produce a stretch, for example, bouncing. Static stretching is far more effective and less likely to cause injury.
★ Pay particular attention to the muscle groups or limbs you are about to exercise.
★ Stretch only to a point where you feel tension, but not pain.
★ Hold each stretch for between ten to thirty seconds.
★ Don't hold your breath – remember to breathe and take deep slow breaths!

Cooling down: this is just as important as warming up. A gradual easing off at the end of your exercise programme helps the circulation to remove any unwanted waste products, such as lactic acid, from the muscles and helps to prevent stiffness and soreness the next day.

A good stretch!

1. QUADS STRETCH Stand side-ways next to a firm support or wall which you can hold on to for balance if necessary. Stand straight and keep your tummy tucked in throughout the exercise. Bend your right leg at the knee so that your foot comes up to or touches your bottom and hold it in position with your right hand gripping the front of your ankle. You should feel the stretch running along the front of your thigh. Hold for ten seconds and repeat with the other leg.

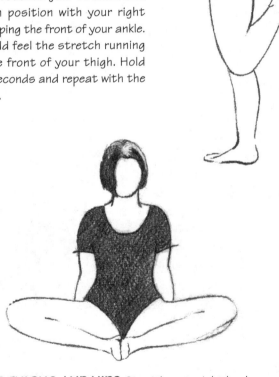

2. INNER THIGHS AND HIPS Sit with a straight back, your legs bent at the knees and your soles of your feet touching. Keep your tummy tucked in and gently allow your knees to fall to the floor so that you feel the stretch on the inside of your thighs. Hold for ten seconds and repeat.

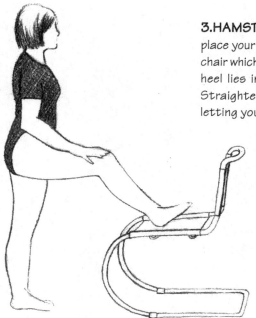

3.HAMSTRINGS Standing straight, place your right heel on the seat of a chair which is positioned so that your heel lies in the middle of the seat. Straighten the leg slowly by gently letting your knee face back towards the floor until you feel the stretch on the back of the thigh. Hold the stretch for ten seconds and repeat with the other leg.

4. CALVES Face a wall and place both hands at shoulder-height flat against it. You should be far enough away to be able to stand upright while having the arms slightly bent at the elbow. Step back about eighteen inches with your right foot, bending your left knee but keeping your right leg straight. Centre your weight between your legs, using the wall as support and gently push your right heel into the floor. You should feel a stretch along the length of the calf. Hold for ten seconds and repeat on the other side.

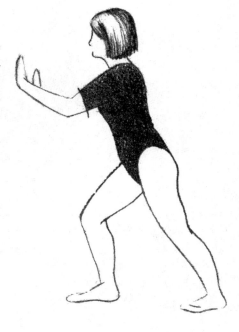

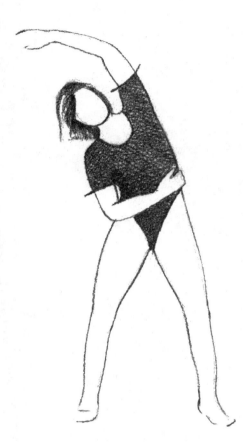

5. SIDE STRETCH Stand with your feet two to three feet apart, your knees slightly bent and your toes pointing slightly outwards. Put your left arm on your hip, raise your right arm to the ceiling with your hand open and gently flex to the side, reaching up as far as possible with your right arm. Stay facing forwards all the time and keep your pelvis still. Hold for a few seconds and repeat on the other side, breathing out as you stretch and in as you straighten.

Immediate benefits of increased activity improve:

★ well-being ★ stamina
★ suppleness ★ tone and posture
★ power ★ strength

Weight loss

As a nation, we have become increasingly inactive. Our energy requirements have fallen from 2400 to 1900 calories a day over the last forty years. No wonder we are getting fatter.

Any attempt to lose weight by changing your diet should be

accompanied by an increase in physical activity. Aerobic exercise is one of the best kinds of exercise for this purpose, but don't be over optimistic about its effect – to lose 500 g (1 lb) of fat you need to burn over 3000 calories. (See table below.)

Nevertheless, a small daily increase in the number of calories you use up each day can have significant effects over a period of time. For example, if you were to walk an extra 1.5 km (a mile) a day, every day, theoretically you would lose approximately 500 g (1 lb) a month.

But it is not just the burning up of calories that will help your weight control. Regular sustained exercise increases the tick-over rate of the body's metabolism which means that it burns more calories even when it is at rest. And don't be put off by thinking that if you exercise you will just eat more and counteract any good you have done. Most people who exercise regularly find that exercise tends to suppress their appetite for an hour or so afterwards.

Calories burnt by an average person exercising for twenty minutes	
Archery	88
Badminton	132
Boxing	302
Canoeing (leisurely)	60
Housework	80
Cooking	64
Cycling	88 @ 8 km/h (5 mph)
	136 @ 16 km/h (10 mph)
Dancing	100
Shopping	84
Football	180
Heavy gardening	150 to 200
Golf	116
Ironing	40 to 80
Sitting quietly	28
Swimming	100 to 230
Tennis	148
Walking at 6 km/h (4 mph)	110

Prescribing exercise

For years GPs have been advising their patients to do some exercise. And, for just as long, the advice has fallen on deaf ears. Now a new scheme whereby GPs are joining forces with local leisure centres or, in some cases, actually setting up their own gyms, is really taking off. Although these schemes are still being evaluated, there is no doubt about the benefits. Some GPs already report a decrease in the amount of drugs they prescribe – particularly hypertensive and diabetic medication.

I am all for this idea. My only concern is that patients should not see it as a one-off six-month or a year's course only. I cannot stress often enough that we should all be aiming for a long-term change in our levels of activity.

Seeking medical advice

It goes without saying that anyone with a medical condition, such as asthma or diabetes, should seek their doctor's advice before embarking on a programme.

It is also a good idea for men over forty-five and women over fifty, who have not seen their doctor for a while, to pop in and let the doctor know what they are planning to do. It is a useful opportunity for the doctor to check blood pressure and answer any specific queries. Most adults, however, do not need to see a doctor before becoming physically active.

As a general rule, you should never exercise or push yourself if you have a cold or infection.

ARE YOU PREGNANT?

Any exercise a women does during pregnancy will depend very much on her level of activity before she became pregnant. It is certainly not the time to embark on a new exercise programme. In the absence of any problems, there is no reason why most women cannot continue existing patterns of exercise – at least up until the last couple of months and, in some cases, right up until delivery. (Many exercises, of course, are impossible at this stage!) The exceptions are contact sports, plus horse-riding and skiing, which carry a risk of falls.

There is a school of thought that says exercise in the first twelve weeks of pregnancy may increase your chances of miscarriage. It is not a view I subscribe to, but if any woman has bleeding or pain during this time then I would advise her to give exercise a miss until it settles down.

Exercise and osteoporosis

As we get older our bones tend to get thinner and more brittle. In one in ten men, and one in three women over the age of fifty the bones can become so thin that they collapse and fracture – a condition called osteoporosis. This also leads to loss of height as the spine crumbles; pain; deformity (the dowager's hump); and fractures of the hip and wrist following the slightest knock or fall.

Bone is a living tissue and responds to the stresses and strains that are put upon it. The less active you are, the thinner your bones will be. Now that many of us live into our eighties, it is important that we keep our bones as healthy as possible by remaining active.

All types of exercise help in this, but the best forms are those which are weight bearing (in other words, those where you have to stand up as opposed to non-weight bearing exercises such as cycling and swimming).

Osteoporosis is a particular problem in post-menopausal women. There is also an inevitable decrease in the strength of all our bones as we get older. The stronger they are when we hit our fifties the less likely they are to develop osteoporosis. Another very good reason for being active throughout life.

✉ Useful addresses

▶ Arthritis Care, 18 Stephenson Way, London NW1 2HD. Telephone: 0171 916 1500. Free helpline: 0800 289170.

▶ British Heart Foundation, The, 14 Fitzhardinge Street, London W1H 4DH. Telephone: 0171 935 0185.

▶ Exercise Association, The, Unit 4, Angel Gate, City Road, London EC1V 2PT. Telephone: 0171 278 0811. Information on exercise available.

▶ National Osteoporosis Society, PO Box 10, Radstock, Bath BA3 3YB. Telephone: 01761 471771. Send an sae for leaflets and more information.

▶ National Sports Medicine Institute, St Bartholemew's Medical College, Charterhouse Square, London EC1M 6BQ. Telephone: 0171 251 0583.

▶ Research into Ageing, 15–17 St Cross Street, London EC1N 8UN. Telephone: 0171 404 6878.

▶ Sports Council, The, 16 Upper Woburn Place, London WC1H 0QP. Telephone: 0171 388 1277.

CHAPTER THREE

'DOES THAT MOLE LOOK FUNNY TO YOU?'

★ Vitamin A and C are important for a healthy complexion.

★ Drinking fresh water helps keep the skin moist.

★ Seek medical advice for skin problems such as acne, rosacea, eczema and psoriasis. Doctors do take these seriously.

★ The sun is the major cause of skin cancer and of premature ageing. For an all-year tan, use fake tans.

★ Poor diet, smoking and consuming alcohol all age the skin.

★ Learn the signs of skin cancer.

MONDAY'S CHOICE

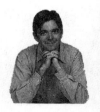

Great Skin

Skin is the body's front-line defence against the world, but in most people's minds skin care is associated with vanity and endless hours spent pampering it with various creams, lotions and splashes in front of a mirror, and is rarely thought to be a health issue. Having said that, most people also regard a flawless skin as a sign of good health, and it is often one of the first things people look at. Considering skin from a health point of view – particularly ways of looking after it – certainly makes good sense and that is why I have devoted a chapter to it.

Good diet and nutrition have a profound effect on the appearance of skin.

Skin problems, in fact, are surprisingly common. About one in five people have a skin condition during their lifetime, and one in eight of my surgery hours – and most other GPs' – are devoted to dealing with them.

In addition to being painful and irritating, skin conditions can have devastating psychological consequences. Sadly, sufferers are often made to feel like social lepers – especially in swimming pools. Nobody should ever underestimate how demoralising a chronic skin condition can be, particularly if it is plainly visible for all to see.

For the most part, I will be discussing general ways to keep skin healthy and youthful, but I will also touch upon a few of the more common skin diseases.

By skin care, I do not mean advice about which moisturiser or face pack to use. It is no good spending a fortune on the latest skin care products if we fail to appreciate that what we eat and drink, and how much we smoke, affects the way our skin looks and feels. It is crucial to understand the effect these influences have because true and effective skin care comes from within as well as from without.

This brings me to the worst culprit when it comes to skin damage – exposure to sunlight. Not only does the sun cause premature ageing of the skin – which is why exposed parts of the body, such as hands, face and neck, look so much older than the covered parts – it also causes skin cancer, the second most common cancer in the UK.

Latest figures show there are 40 000 new cases of skin cancer diagnosed each year – an alarming eighty-four per cent increase in the last ten years. Although much is blamed on the thinning ozone layer, this particular effect is negligible compared with the modern obsession with a 'healthy' tan – and the resulting fondness for holidays spent basking in the sun.

Up until the beginning of this century tans were associated, for example, with peasants and other forms of outdoor work and thought to be 'common' – vulgar. It was not until the 1920s, when Coco Chanel popularised the tanned look, that it became fashionable. Despite the interest in a pale complexion in the 1990s, it is unlikely that this will really catch on. The damage has been done. People like being tanned and now associate it with feeling and looking more attractive.

Many dermatologists say that there is no such thing as a safe tan and that we should all avoid the sun. I do not think this is realistic advice. I, too, enjoy being brown. However, as a doctor, I know there are some common sense ways of going about tanning which reduce the risks.

Also, as a doctor, I am fed up with people being taken in by the many pseudo-scientific claims that are made for skin-care products. I can understand that the beautifully made up youthful lady selling the latest 'revolutionary' anti-ageing product is much more convincing than a fuddy-duddy doctor saying that soap and water are the only things you need, but the truth is that there is rarely any scientific evidence to back up the former's hard sell. So, in this chapter, I will also mention some of the latest products on the market, and discuss whether I think it is worth parting with your money or not.

Skin – the facts

The skin is made up of cells arranged in two layers:

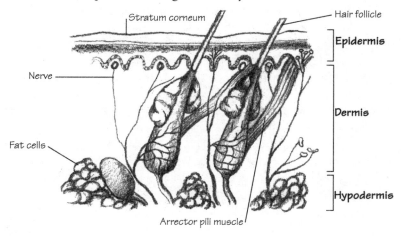

The epidermis – the top layer of skin – is as thick as a sheet of writing paper. Its outer layer is made up entirely of dead, dehydrated, flattened cells, called the stratum corneum, which form the body's main protective barrier, preventing water loss and infection. These cells slough off when we wash and when the skin rubs against clothing. The lower layer is made up of living cells which reproduce themselves every three to six weeks. Each new cell pushes the old one further away from the supply of nutrients and thus produces a layer of dead cells.

The dermis is many times thicker and is a living tissue supplied with small blood vessels and nerves. Sweat glands, sebaceous glands and hair follicles punctuate the skin at regular intervals. Sweat glands help regulate body temperature and the sebaceous glands produce an oily secretion which serves as a waterproof layer. The bulk of the dermis is made up of stretchy fibres of collagen and elastic, which form the skeleton of the skin and are therefore crucial in the ageing process. The subcutaneous fatty tissue acts as a heat insulator and a further protective layer.

Diet and skin

Diet and good nutrition have a profound effect on the appearance of skin. Like any other organ, skin needs nutrients to maintain its normal healthy function and some of it, such as the face and hands, is on show for all to see.

A diet rich in vitamins A and C is important for a healthy complexion. Both are antioxidants (vitamins which are believed to help us live longer and look younger) and protect us against the ravages of pollution, ultraviolet light and cigarette smoke. Vitamin C is also essential for the healthy production of collagen, which is the main architectural support in the skin.

Fluid intake also has an effect on the skin's appearance. Drinking plenty of fresh water helps to keep the skin moist and plumps out fine lines and wrinkles. It also helps to maintain circulation of both blood and tissue fluids which ensure an adequate supply of nutrients and oxygen, and helps to wash away any waste products produced by all living cells.

As a general guideline, we should drink 1.75–2.25 litres (3–4 pints) of fresh water a day. This may seem like a large quantity, but when you consider that our bodies are over half water (65% for men, 55% for women), it begins to make sense.

SMOKING

When it comes to ageing, smoking is one of the worst enemies of the skin – second only to harmful exposure to the sun. Smoking ages the skin in a number of ways. Firstly, it interferes with the skin's blood circulation, decreasing the amount of nutrients and oxygen the skin receives, as well as allowing waste products to build up, often giving the skin a greyish tinge.

In addition, and more long term, smoking actually destroys the collagen fibres – the skin's main structural support. Studies suggest that benzene-related chemicals in cigarette smoke destroy hydrogen bonds and thus weaken the collagen in the skin, promoting wrinkles.

Another unsightly consequence of smoking is the large open facial pores, which are found either side of the nose and under the eyes. Smokers often have darker rings under their eyes than non-smokers and look older.

Alcohol

Oscar Wilde said that every glass of wine leaves its mark on a face and sadly he was not far from the truth. Alcohol has both short- and long-term effects on the skin.

In the short term it dilates blood vessels and leads to a flushed complexion. Long-term drinking then makes some of these changes permanent, as well as thickening the skin and giving it an unhealthy sheen. The only way to avoid such damage is to stick within the sensible drinking guidelines (see Chapter Seven).

Do not, however, confuse a heavy drinker's complexion with a skin condition called rosacea (see below). Although this can be made worse by drinking, it is not caused by alcohol and can be treated.

Rosacea: this skin condition affects one in fifteen people and is caused by an abnormality of the skin over the nose, cheeks, chin and forehead. At first, sufferers notice that these areas tend to flush very easily, particularly in hot environments, and after eating spicy foods and drinking alcohol. The latter leads to many rosacea sufferers being wrongly labelled as heavy drinkers.

Sadly, a lot of people with this condition are unaware that it is treatable. Simple antibiotics, both in tablet and cream form, can have good effects. If left untreated rosacea invariably worsens leading to permanent facial redness and, in really severe cases, particularly in men, may lead to a disfiguring overgrowth of the skin on the nose (rhinophyma).

Natural ageing

However well we care for our skin, there are some inevitable changes dictated by time and other factors over which we have no control.

Infancy: collagen fibres are at their most plentiful in infancy and are responsible for the characteristic supple smooth appearance of infant skin. However, the skin is thin and the sebaceous glands underdeveloped, which means it is also highly sensitive and easily irritated.

Teenagers: hormonal changes during teenage years mean that the skin tends to produce a greater amount of sebum (the skin's natural protective oil) than older skins, making it oily and coarser-looking. This excess oil also makes teenagers more prone to spots (see Acne, page 99). Cleansing to remove the build-up of dirt and grease is the most important aspect of skin care during this time.

Cleansing to remove the build-up of dirt and grease is the most important aspect of skin care during teenage years.

Adults: skin becomes thinner with age, and the main difference between men and women is that women's skin is thinner and less greasy than men's. Unfair, perhaps, but this means that women are more susceptible to changes associated with ageing.

Ageing also brings changes in the 'mechanical' properties of the skin. Older skin feels drier and tends to be scaly in the elderly. These changes, of course, can also occur during cold weather or low humidity, and central heating certainly does not help.

Twenty-year-olds: the hormones of twenty-year-olds are still settling down and oil glands are still active, so spots can continue to be a problem. But it is also the time when skin is at its most resilient and elastic. The first signs of ageing may become apparent in our late twenties, usually around the eyes as the skin is thinner there than elsewhere.

Thirty-year-olds: in this age group, the skin produces less sebum and skin lipids, which leads to dryness. This is accelerated by any outdoor lifestyle that exposes the skin to wind, water and sun. The skin continues to get drier as we age and leads to the appearance of fine lines. Wrinkles may start to appear as the skin's elasticity and firmness decline. Wrinkling of the skin is also caused by exposure to the sun (see Ageing in the sun, below). Melanin production also changes and can lead to uneven pigmentation. The rate at which epidermis cells divide and reproduce leads to a relatively thinner skin in old age. At the same time, the ability of the skin to repair itself slows down.

Forties to fifties: the loss of elasticity and changes in collagen, mean the signs of ageing become more obvious. The skin is thinner and surface lines are deeper. The skin produces very little natural oil. In our fifties, lines and wrinkles are more established and the skin becomes drier. The supporting dermal layer loses its tone causing a gradual sagging and wrinkling. In addition, the mechanical action of fifty years of facial movements start to take their toll.

Sixties-plus: in the ten years following the menopause, women lose about thirty per cent of collagen as a result of oestrogen deficiency. The skin becomes noticeably thinner. There is some evidence that hormone replacement therapy (HRT) can help maintain healthier skin. Recent research has also shown that oestrogen creams can make skin appear more youthful, but as oestrogen is a prescription-only drug it cannot be included in cosmetic face creams.

Ageing in the sun

The sun, as I have said already, is the skin's worst enemy. It is singlehandedly responsible for up to ninety-five per cent of our facial ageing or, as dermatologists are fond of saying, 'Years do not cause skin damage. It's the number of summers you put yourself through.'

Without sunlight, we probably would not get serious wrinkles until we were in our sixth or seventh decade of life.

Photoageing: If we took skin from the buttocks of an eighty-year-old woman who had never exposed her bottom to the sun, it would be as smooth as the face of a thirty-year-old, with only a slight loss in elasticity. Photoageing – as this type of ageing is known – is the reason why our faces, hands and necks go wrinkly, but not the rest of our bodies. Without sunlight, we probably would not get serious wrinkles until we were in our sixth or seventh decade of life.

Photodamage describes the chronic structural damage to skin caused by long-term exposure to sun. In photodamaged skin, the epidermis is much thinner, the melanocytes (cells) decrease in places and become more active in others, and there are also some deep structural changes.

Sunlight can penetrate into the dermis and destroy the structural supports of the skin – the collagen and elastic fibres. This means the outer layer sinks into the ridges and folds of the inner layer, and forms wrinkles. Wrinkling, however, is not the only effect of the sun on the skin. Differences in pigmentation – brown spots – also occur as a result of damage to pigment cells in sun-exposed skin. Broken veins can also occur because the blood vessels in damaged skin are not well supported, allowing them to widen and become visible on the skin's surface.

UVA and UVB: It is the ultraviolet component of light – made of ultraviolet A (UVA) and ultraviolet B (UVB) – that is responsible for photoageing.

UVA light is present in the atmosphere all year. It is highly penetrative and can travel through clothing, glass, water and clouds, and passes deep into the skin destroying its support network of collagen and elastin. It is responsible for premature ageing, and long-term exposure to its rays leads to wrinkles, brown spots and broken blood vessels. It is also linked with at least one type of skin cancer.

UVB rays only present a problem when the sun is actually shining because they are easily blocked by clouds, clothing, glass and water and when they do get through only penetrate the upper layers of the skin. They are responsible for tanning by stimulating melanocytes (cells) into producing the pigment melanin. Too much UVB results in sunburn and is a major cause of skin cancer. UVB also speeds up cell production in the upper layer of the skin, causing it to thicken and take on a leathery texture. The word tan is derived from the Latin for leather.

The right exposure: I am not suggesting that we should never go out in the sun. I like being out in the sun as much as anybody else, but there are sensible and safe ways of going about it.

The first thing to understand is that prolonged sunbathing will not result in a darker or better tan because tanning is a result of the stimulation of the melanocytes (cells) – and these can only produce melanin (pigment) at a certain rate. Increasing your exposure above the amount needed to achieve this stimulation just leads to sunburn not a better tan.

Research suggests that twenty minutes exposure is all that unprotected skin needs to achieve maximum melanin (pigment) production. Sunbathing for any longer than this at any one time has little effect on the speed of tanning, but markedly increases the chances of sunburn, skin damage and cancer. Sunburn is the body's reaction to damage caused by ultraviolet light, and is a sign that we have been over exposed.

Many things influence the amount of ultraviolet radiation reaching the surface of the earth, and it is certainly worth bearing the following points in mind:

The lower a place is relative to sea level, the less UVB penetrates. For example, at the Dead Sea in Israel – 400 m (1312 ft) below sea level – a lot of the burning potential of UVB has been filtered out. Conversely, the higher you are the greater is the risk of burning. We can expect a four per cent increase in the sunburning effect for each 300 m (984 ft) we are above sea level, so mountain climbers should be extra careful.

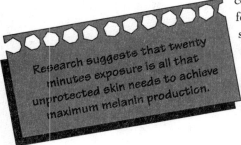

Research suggests that twenty minutes exposure is all that unprotected skin needs to achieve maximum melanin production.

Latitude also makes a difference. The nearer we are to the equator the hotter the sun is.

Time of the year and day is also

important. In the Northern hemisphere the amount of ultraviolet light is 130 times greater in summer than in the middle of the winter, and higher at noon than in the morning.

Cloud cover and pollution also reduce the intensity of the rays reaching the surface of the earth, but do not be lulled into a false sense of security on a cloudy or pollution-hazy day, you can still get sunburned.

Surfaces that reflect light, such as water or snow, increase the amount of ultraviolet light reaching the body. This is why it is so easy to become sunburned when skiing, when on the beach or in the water.

Vitiligo: this skin disease, which Michael Jackson claims to have, is when the melanocytes (skin cells) suddenly stop working. The affected areas then become white and are particularly sensitive to exposure to the sun.

GETTING A HEALTHY TAN

Your skin's ability to tan depends on the amount of melanin (pigment) it contains. This, in turn, depends on genes – as anyone of Celtic ancestry will be aware – and the amount of exposure to the sun. Melanin is black and the colour black absorbs the sun's rays. It is produced in skin cells, called melanocytes, and the pigment is then carried upwards by the epidermal cells and eventually sloughed off at the surface. Getting a healthy tan is dependent on the following:

★ Avoid sunbathing between 11 a.m. and 3 p.m., when the sun is at its strongest. Instead, have a long lunch in the shade or a siesta.

★ Don't spend more than twenty minutes, each side, in the sun without sun-screen protection which contains both UVA and UVB screens.

★ UVB protection: the sun protection factor (SPF) enables you to be exposed to the sun for longer without burning. For example, if your skin begins to redden after ten minutes when unprotected, an SPF15 cream will protect you for fifteen times as long, that is 150 minutes before you burn. Never use a sunscreen with an SPF factor of less than six to eight. ▷

◁ ★ UVA protection is indicated by a star symbol usually shown on the back of the bottle. The protection level is expressed as a fraction of the SPF (sun protection factor). One star means it offers a quarter as much protection against UVA as it does against UVB; and three stars offers three-quarters the protection. Always use a sunscreen that has at least a three-star UVA rating.

★ Take care when bathing near water, sand or concrete. All these reflect and intensify the amount of sunlight you are exposed to.

★ Men with bald heads need to be particularly careful with their scalp, ears and neck.

★ Always moisturise your skin after you have been in the sun. This helps to replenish some of the moisture the skin has lost during the day and can soothe sunburn. Ordinary moisturisers are as good as the more expensive specialist products.

Babies and children

Babies under twelve months old should be kept out of direct sunlight altogether.

Babies under twelve months old should be kept out of direct sunlight altogether, and I can see no earthly reason why parents should want young children to get a tan. Children's skin is highly susceptible to ultraviolet damage, and recent evidence suggests that just one episode of severe sunburn in childhood can predispose a child to skin cancer later in life.

So, if children are exposed to sun, plaster them with a high-factor suncream, for example SPF 20, UVA ***, as well as making sure they wear a T-shirt and sunhat at all times. Remain aware, however, that a T-shirt, particularly when it is wet, may have an SPF (sun protective factor) as low as ten.

When children are in and out of the water, make sure that a waterproof suncream is applied regularly, and keep them out of the sun between 11a.m. and 3 p.m. As a father of two, I know this is not always simple, but it is necessary. It is a routine worth getting into at the start of your holiday.

SUN BEDS

These were once regarded as the safer alternative to sunbathing because they use only UVA rays (see Ageing in the sun, page 91). Recently, however, there have been reports of skin cancer that can only have been caused by sun beds, and some dermatologists now claim that they may be more dangerous than sunbathing.

Although the UVB rays, which cause sunburn, have been filtered out of the light emitted by the fluorescent tubes, the UVA levels are many times higher than that of natural sunlight. These artificially boosted levels far exceed our natural exposure to UVA and can cause premature ageing, abnormal skin colouring and skin cancer.

In addition, dermatologists think the damage caused by sunbathing is cumulative. In other words, all year round use of sun beds may be much more of a problem than sunbathing on an annual holiday. Under-sixteens should not use sun beds. Likewise, people with skin conditions that are made worse by the sun, for example polymorphic light eruption (also known as sun allergy) should never use a sun bed unless under medical direction.

If you are undeterred by all the warnings given above and really cannot resist using a sun bed, then take the following advice:

★ Always use a solarium that is a member of the Association of Sun Tanning Operators. These establishments have agreed a Code of Practice, drawn up by the Health and Safety Executive.
★ Do not put on any make-up or perfume before a sun-bed session.
★ Always wear goggles to protect your eyes.
★ Be extra specially careful if you are fair skinned and burn easily.
★ Do not indulge in more than twenty to thirty sessions a year.

Tanning from a tube or bottle

Strictly speaking this is the only absolutely safe way to get a tan. Although the early products turned people an unattractive streaky orange, there are now some increasingly sophisticated types on the market. Most of these

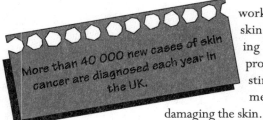

More than 40 000 new cases of skin cancer are diagnosed each year in the UK.

work by simply staining the skin, but there is also increasing interest in developing products which, like real tans, stimulate the production of melanin (pigment) without damaging the skin.

But always remember that the application of fake tans offers no protection against natural ultraviolet rays. You must always continue to protect yourself when exposed to sunlight, and this remains necessary even when you have a deep 'tan'.

Skin cancer – the facts

There are now more than 40 000 new cases of skin cancer diagnosed each year in the UK. The most deadly form, melanoma, causes 1200 deaths a year. Other forms are responsible for more than 500 deaths. There are three types of skin cancer.

Basal cell carcinomas are the commonest. These develop as a small, slow-growing, pearly edged lump or sore. Untreated, they can crust, ulcerate and bleed. They are unique among cancerous tumours in that they do not spread to other parts of the body. They are easier to treat when detected early, and can be cured.

Squamous cell carcinomas are less common, but more dangerous because they can spread to other parts of the body. They usually occur on the face or hands, and develop as a scaling red area which can also bleed easily and ulcerate.

Malignant melanoma is the rarest, but most serious type of cancer. These usually start as small brown or black moles. People at greatest risk include those with a high number of moles or freckles, red or fair hair, blue eyes, and people who do not tan easily or burn in the sun.

A recent study in the *British Medical Journal* found that asking people to count the number of moles on their chest could help them to predict their own risk of melanoma. High mole counts, particularly on the trunk (that is more than seven which measure 2 mm / ¹⁄₁₆ inch or more) were more sensitive and an early indication of potential future problems.

There are a number of things to be on the alert for:

★ Any new mole, particularly on the soles or palms and under the nails.
★ Increasing size: ordinary moles do not change size.
★ A change in shape: typically the edges become irregular and blurred and lose definition.
★ Colour: most melanomas show a lot of pigment variation, and are a mixture of brown and black or red.
★ Inflammation.
★ Crusting or bleeding.
★ Itch: this is a common symptom of melanomas, but ordinary moles can also itch.
★ Small brown changes around the edge: these could be satellite lesions.

If you notice any of the above changes, it is essential to check them out with your doctor.

Other sun-related problems

In addition to sunburn and the danger of contracting skin cancer, up to twenty per cent of the population suffer abnormal skin reactions when exposed to the sun. These are known as photodermatoses.

Polymorphic light eruption (PLE): also known as sun allergy, is the most common. It appears as an itchy rash (for example, prickly heat rash) usually on parts of the body, such as the leg, arms and chest that are covered in winter but exposed in summer. I suffered from prickly heat rash for twenty plus years and it ruined many a good holiday. Fortunately, most cases of prickly heat are due to the UVA portion of sunlight, and the advent of modern sunscreens has transformed my holidays. The old-fashioned UVB screens in suntanning products made matters worse by giving a false sense of security while offering no protection against the troublesome UVA components. Since using a UVA sunscreen, I have not had a single attack of prickly heat.

Herpes – cold sores: can be brought on by exposure to the sun and also cold weather, which is why they are a problem for skiers. Total sunblock, worn on and around the lips, can prevent these breaking out.

Eczema and psoriasis

The sun is good news for some skin problems – eczema and psoriasis, for example, can improve in sunny weather but it is still important to wear adequate protection. People with a sensitive skin should make sure they use an hypoallergenic non-perfumed sunscreen. A pharmacist will advise.

Acne and spots

Acne is a condition that affects the parts of the skin that have a high number of oil-producing sebaceous glands, namely the face, back and chest. These glands are under the control of the sex hormones, which is why the onset of acne most commonly coincides with puberty. Spots form when pores clog up with oil and skin debris.

Acne usually first occurs in the early teen years, and is often at its worst between the ages of seventeen and nineteen. It gradually improves from the early twenties, although it can persist up to the age of forty. None of us, of course, is immune from the odd pimple every now and again.

One common myth is that chocolate causes spots – none of my patients believes me when I tell them this is untrue, but there is absolutely no evidence that there is a link.

People with spots need to be meticulous about skin care. Pharmacies sell a host of skin washes and lotions which can provide good basic protection against acne. Make sure you follow the pharmacist's advice and do not be misled by advertisements that claim this or that product can cure spots in a matter of days.

Unfortunately, not all people respond to this type of treatment, so please do not hesitate to ask your GP for help. Doctors do not have any magical remedies, but we do take the condition seriously and have a lot of effective prescription-only treatments we can suggest.

One interesting advance is the use of zinc supplements. Some studies have shown that taking doses of elemental zinc, for example, 50 mg daily for six to twelve weeks can help.

To squeeze or not to squeeze is an issue which many doctors and beauticians disagree about. Doctors believe the best way to deal with a spot is to keep the skin clean and fingers off. Dabbing with an antiseptic may also help. To be realistic, however, no one likes to walk around with a 'ripe' spot on their face. If you really cannot leave it alone, read the following list first:

For more information, contact the Acne Support Group (see Useful addresses on page 104).

Skin-care products

We spend an amazing £446 million a year on skin-care products. Prime users are women aged between thirty and fifty years, but a growing number of men are now falling for the clever advertising and marketing hype. Are we getting value for money or simply being blinded by science?

It is only too easy to be fooled into thinking that the more you spend on skin-care products the more you are going to get for your money, and the more attractive you will look as a result. But in reality the biggest difference between a really expensive so-called anti-ageing product and a pot of E45 cream is, probably, the price.

★ Squeezing a spot will increase the surrounding inflammation, attract more attention and increase the chances of scarring.

★ If you must squeeze, do this only when the head is yellow.

★ Be particularly careful about hygiene – always wash your hands before and after touching a spot.

★ Do not continue to squeeze until the spot bleeds. This will increase the chances of scarring.

Moisturisers: anti-ageing products are basically moisturisers. Water in skin gives the complexion a fresh healthy look, but, as it ages, skin is less able to retain moisture. When the skin loses moisture – particularly during winter when the air is drier – it becomes dry and cracked. Facial skin loses more than 1.2 litres (2 pints) of water a month.

All moisturisers are essentially water in an emulsion of oil, which enables the skin temporarily to trap water. This can improve your skin – making it shinier and puffier, which reduces wrinkles – but for the same effect you will need to moisturise your skin whenever it is dry. Wrinkles and fine lines are the direct result of dryness, so moisturisers do help. All moisturising products do this whether cheap or expensive.

Anti-ageing products, then, are really just expensive moisturisers. Dermatologists say that the only true anti-ageing ingredients that these products contain is sunscreen. And remember you have to apply your sunscreen many times during the course of a day to benefit and remain constantly protected.

Other wheezes that are used to justify the inflated prices of anti-ageing products are the inclusion of collagen and elastin. But, while no doctor would deny these are essential components of skin itself, there is no evidence that skin can make use of these when they are applied externally.

AHAs: the recently introduced AHAs (alpha hydroxy acids) have caught on in a big way. These are basically naturally occurring acids which work like a mild exfoliating agent, speeding up skin-cell turnover. This means they get rid of old dry skin cells of the stratum corneum to reveal newer fresher ones. There is no doubt that, in the short term, they can make a difference to the appearance of your skin but I cannot help thinking that this layer is there for a purpose and it may not be a good idea to remove it. Removing it may even make ageing more likely in the long term.

Vitamin-enriched products: another recent innovation has been the move to leap on the antioxidant bandwagon. The rationale is that the skin is the last organ to benefit from the vitamins we eat and that we can make sure it gets enough by using vitamin-enriched creams. Vitamin E is the most popular and many creams are now marketed on this fact. However what you do not hear in the slick sales talk is that vitamin E has been used for ages to stop such creams going rancid. In other words, it is a preservative. There is absolutely no proof it will help keep skin youthful. Yes, antioxidants are important but the best way to benefit from them is to eat a healthy diet.

Prescription-only products: The only true anti-ageing products are treatments for photodamaged skin that are only available on prescription. Most are derivatives of vitamin A and there is some evidence they can improve wrinkles, mottling and skin roughness. They were introduced in the early 1970s for the treatment of acne, and there is also some evidence that they are effective for repairing sun-damaged skin. Any improvements, however, only occur after several months – nine months for best effect – of continuous use of the products. They are believed to work by penetrating deep into the skin and activating fibre cells. They reduce the number of fine lines, decrease patchy skin pigmentation and improve skin colour. However, like all drugs, they cause side-effects – mainly skin irritation.

There is only one product (Retinova) licensed for this type of usage which contains the vitamin A derivative, tretinoin, and it is a prescription-only drug.

Skin cleansing

The build-up of pollutants, make-up and dead skin cells on the skin's surface may increase the chances of spots and give the skin a dull appearance. The natural turnover of skin cells is twenty days, but cleansing and scrubbing (exfoliating) can increase this to fourteen days.

When washing your face make sure the water is warm rather than hot and always rinse with cold clean water afterwards.

There is no need to use fancy expensive products. Soap and water are fine for most types of skin. Those with dry skin, however, should avoid soap-based products and just use water or a non-soap cream cleanser.

When washing your face make sure the water is warm rather than hot and always rinse with cold clean water afterwards.

DRY SKIN

This can be a problem, particularly in late winter when the air is drier and more water tends to be lost from the skin. Cold weather, heavy colds and central heating all have a dehydrating effect on the skin.

People with eczema are particularly prone to dry skin, and good basic skin care and moisturising can help keep eczema under control. If you are prone to dry skin:

★ Avoid soap and bubble baths.
★ Never wash your hair in the bath – the shampoo can have a drying effect on the skin of the rest of your body.
★ Men should avoid using aftershaves and colognes on their face, and women should make sure they use hypoallergenic cosmetics.
★ Moisturise your skin using a non-perfumed cheap hypoallergenic moisturiser at least twice a day or after every time you bathe or wash your face.

Facial massage

This is very good for the skin. Indeed, one of the problems in evaluating new skin-care products is that it is hard to distinguish between the effects of the massage and the benefits of the cream that is used for the massage.

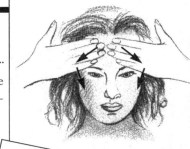

Massage improves the blood supply to the face which means a better supply of oxygen and the quicker removal of waste products. It also improves the circulation of the lymphatic system which is the body's natural draining system for fluid surrounding the tissues.

The skin should be massaged

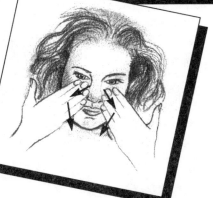

using light pressure, and downward flowing movements of the hands. Stroking, patting and rolling the skin is also beneficial.

Plastic surgery

I can understand why some people want to resort to plastic surgery, but I always advise my patients against it.

The first thing to appreciate is that you are getting into a vicious circle – the effects are short-lived. Even the best facelift rarely lasts more than a few years. So, the moment you have the first facelift you are tying yourself into a life-long commitment to repeat the process. Once you have started, you are on a very expensive conveyor belt.

You also have to bear in mind that standards vary tremendously. Most cosmetic surgery is only available in the private sector, but I always strongly recommend my patients never to use a cosmetic surgeon unless he or she is employed as an NHS consultant in cosmetic surgery, and is a member of an approved body such as the British Association of Aesthetic Plastic Surgeons (see useful addresses below) which will provide a list of members on request.

✉ Useful addresses

▶ Acne Support Group, PO Box 230, Hayes, Middlesex UB4 9HW. Telephone: 0181 561 6868 (ansaphone during evenings).

▶ Beauty Care and Cosmetic Camouflage Service, The British Red Cross Society, 9 Grosvenor Crescent, London SW1X 7EJ. Telephone: 0171 235 5454.

▶ National Eczema Society, 163 Eversholt Street, London NW1 1BU. Telephone: 0171 388 4097.

▶ Psoriasis Association, 7 Milton Street, Northampton NN2 7JG. Telephone: 01604 711129.

▶ British Association of Aesthetic Plastic Surgeons, c/o Royal College of Surgeons, 35-43 Lincoln's Inn Fields, London WC2A 3PN. Telephone: 0171 405 2234.

▶ The Vitiligo Society, 19 Fitzroy Square London W1P 5HQ. Telephone: 0171 388 8905.

CHAPTER FOUR

'I'M NOT WAVING, I'M DROWNING'

★ Never underestimate the power of relaxation.

★ Be realistic about what you can do.

★ Spend an hour a day enjoying yourself.

★ Learn to say no.

★ Tell someone how you feel.

★ Never neglect exercise.

★ Eat healthily.

TUESDAY'S CHOICE

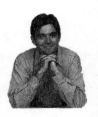

Less Stress

Stress is one of those words we use on an almost casual daily basis, yet few of us really know or understand what it means. This is not surprising because stress is actually very hard to define, and is really an umbrella term for a host of emotions, including anxiety, tension, exhaustion, panic, unhappiness and insecurity.

Ask anyone what causes stress and you will get an endless list of things which are an inevitable part of day-to-day life in the 1990s: bereavement, a messy divorce, moving house, pressures at work, examination results, financial worries, redundancy, unemployment, bullying, domestic violence and abuse. The common factor in all these events is that they are often out of our control – and that is why they are stressful. But while stress itself may be inevitable, getting stressed does not have to be.

It is not so much the events that are the problem, but the way we react to them. It all comes back to the insecurity and panic we experience when we perceive life and other people to be out of our control. As soon as we feel that we are losing control, we succumb to stress and its related problems – physical illnesses, emotional imbalance, even mental disorders.

One study which illustrated this and changed the way many doctors thought of stress was the Whitehall study of civil servants. Doctors monitored the incidence of heart attacks and other stress-related problems in thousands of civil servants at different stages of the career ladder.

The study's first findings made a mockery of the conventional wisdom that it is high-powered executives who are at the highest risk of stress-related problems and illnesses. People in the lowest civil-servant grade were discovered to be at higher risk. The risk then diminished with each step up the career ladder. When these findings were studied in more detail two things became evident – lack of support from family, friends or colleagues, and lack of control over one's life, are very important in determining whether a person is susceptible to stress.

The executive may have more demands made upon him or her and more responsibility to cope with, but it is not the demands *per se* that damage health, but demands partnered by lack of control – this is stress.

This also highlights the fact that stress has its positive side and can be good for us. For example, it can be a motivator which pushes us on to achieve greater things than we would have done without it. It can keep us going as we strive to get on in life and cope with the various obstacles that are thrown our way. This is why it is so important to distinguish between harmful and good stress, and appreciate, in learning how to manage it, that it can work in our favour.

A healthy lifestyle is even more essential to someone who is stressed than somebody who is not. For this reason every chapter in this book is essential reading. Good diet, for example, is often the first thing to fall by the wayside when a person is under pressure. So be particularly careful to follow the healthy-eating advice in Chapter One.

Sleep problems are also often related to anxiety and stress so, in addition to tackling the cause of the stress-related problem, there are some sensible guidelines you can follow to ensure you get a good night's sleep (see Chapter Six).

Lastly, never neglect exercise (see Chapter Two). You may feel like hunkering down and hiding in a corner when you are stressed, but physical fitness is one of the best ways to avoid brooding, which leads to a build-up of stress and stress-related illness.

Emotional and mental signs of stress

★ Anxiety
★ Tension
★ Panic
★ Edginess
★ Irritability
★ Tearfulness
★ Excessive self-criticism
★ Low self-esteem
★ Increased smoking and alcohol intake
★ Sleep disturbances
★ Loss of appetite
★ Agitation
★ Inability to cope
★ Frustration
★ Depression
★ General malaise

Stress-related factors

Acknowledging that you are suffering from stress is the first and in many ways the hardest step. Many people believe that this very admission is a sign of weakness — an admission they cannot therefore allow and which must be denied at all costs. In truth, nothing can be done until we face the fact that we are stressed. Many of its signs, as you will see from the adjacent list, are easy to spot, and as if that list is not bad

You need to be self-indulgent and put yourself top of the list of your priorities.

enough, the consequences do not end there. Physical symptoms – illnesses of one kind or another – (see below) are also common.

All in the mind?

Many people with stress-related disorders find it hard to believe, or accept, that physical symptoms are due to stress. And, as doctors know too well, it is not unusual when telling a patient that headaches, for example, are stress-related to find the patient thinks we are suggesting that the symptoms are all in the mind. Nothing could be further from the truth. Stress can cause, and worsen, a wide range of physical complaints and symptoms.

Take heartburn or indigestion, both very common physical consequences of stress. One of the body's reactions to stress is to produce more stomach acid. This is as strong as battery acid and, when produced in high quantities, can literally burn away the lining of the stomach making it inflamed and tender (gastritis) – a very real physical illness with very real physical effects that are certainly not in the mind.

All these can be treated with a variety of medication, but it is vital to identify stress as a causative factor. If you do not do anything about the underlying cause, then all you do is cover up the symptoms until the medicines run out and the whole process starts again. It makes sense to face up to what is causing the stress and, whenever possible, allow the body to heal itself. If your GP suggests that stress may be a factor, do take his/her advice seriously: they are not dismissing your symptoms.

Other common stress-related conditions include:

★ Migraine and tension headaches
★ Irritable bowel syndrome
★ Irregular menstruation
★ High blood pressure
★ Palpitations
★ Skin problems
★ Diminished sex drive
★ Impotence
★ Abdominal pain
★ Physical tensions

Who suffers from stress?

Everyone is subjected to stress, but only some of us develop stress-related illness. As I have already said stress is most likely to affect people who have least control over external events, their living and working environment, and destiny. So housewives and factory-floor workers are at greater risk than the company chairman. They are also far less likely to be able to get the help they need. Never belittle the things you have to cope with — even if you are not running a business empire.

EXTERNAL STRESSES

Two American doctors, Holmes and Rahe, have devised what they call a Social Ratings Scale to allow people to assess the rate of external stresses in their lives. To do this, they have ranked more than forty life events (some of which are listed below) according to their potential to cause us stress. Anyone who scores more than 300 units in any one year is considered to have a greatly increased risk of stress-related illnesses. A score of 150 carries only a slight risk.

But, please, only use the following chart has a crude indicator and, above all, at the risk of repeating myself, remember that it is not so much the stress factor itself, but how we react to stress that counts.

Life event	score	Life event	score
Death of partner	100	Gain of new family member	39
Divorce	73	Sexual difficulties	39
Marital separation	65	Change in financial state	38
Death of close family member	63	Major mortgage	32
Personal injury or illness	53	Change in work responsibilities	29
Marriage	50	Son or daughter leaving home	29
Dismissal from work	47	Moving house	20
Retirement	45	Change in eating habits	15
Change in health of family member	44	Holiday	13
Pregnancy	40	Change in schools	20

Children and teenagers

Stress is not just an adult problem, children and teenagers suffer from it too. This is hardly surprising when you consider that all adult stress-related problems – resulting, for example, from bereavement, divorce, moving house, redundancy and unemployment (see table on page 109) – have a very obvious knock-on effect on children.

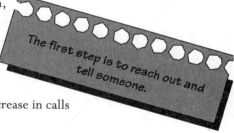

Stress is not just an adult problem, children and teenagers suffer from it too.

In addition, children have their own problems, for example being bullied at school, being the victims of verbal, psychological or physical abuse. Then there are school studies, examination results and peer pressures to contend with.

Some experts believe the problem is exacerbated by the fact that today's youth have become very isolated from their parents; and the extended family of grandparents, aunts, uncles and cousins has become a rarity, as has a father in many instances. Activities have become solitary – watching television, playing computer games, and many children are latchkey children, with a single parent or both parents working. Very early exposure to harmful substances, such as drugs, glue-sniffing and alcohol, or the introduction to sex, and worries about sexual orientation, are now common.

In response to the growing stress levels among children and teenagers, there has been a reemergence of school counsellors. And the British Association of Counselling has reported a recent doubling of stress-related problems in this age group.

The Royal College of Psychiatrists has also recently drawn attention to the fact that depression is a common problem among school-age children, affecting children as young as seven. Symptoms include persistent moodswings, unhappiness, sleep disturbances, aggressive behaviour and excessive worrying.

The first step is to reach out and tell someone.

The Samaritans also report an increase in calls from children and teenagers.

In these circumstances, it is hardly necessary for me to say that children and teenagers, and young people awaiting examination results at school and university, or seeking jobs, are very dependent on adults for help. Being given opportunities to talk to parents, schoolteachers, tutors and, if necessary, a family doctor or counsellor about the pressures and stresses they are experiencing is absolutely vital for their health and general well-being.

Elderly people

Ageing brings its own pressures and stresses, especially for those who are suffering from ill health, financial worries, loneliness, finding it difficult to adjust to retirement, feeling housebound, and even feeling one has out-stayed one's use and welcome.

Many solutions lie in all that is contained in the various chapters of this book. But, having said that, and without wishing to be considered ageist, some elderly people are naturally dependent on the younger and more physically able among us to keep a special eye on their needs and state of mind. Visits, tender loving care and practical help, can go a very long way to transforming the life of another person. At the very least, the family doctor and social services can be alerted and brought into play.

Coping with stress

Once you accept that you are suffering from stress, the next step is to identify what is causing it. This is usually only too apparent, but identifying, acknowledging and accepting it can be therapeutic in itself.

Removing the cause is more easily said than done. Indeed, many people find that there is very little they can do to change or remove the source of a problem, such as being made redundant, which is why they are stressed in the first place. But that is not the same as saying there is nothing we can do about our response to the problem. Even when we cannot change the situation that first 'triggered' the stress, we can accept this as a fact and start work on changing our attitude and approach to the consequences.

You may need help to do this. Talk to family or friends, or get in touch with professional counsellors. Your GP will be able to help with this – and some now employ counsellors within their practice.

The next thing you need to do is to be self-indulgent and put yourself top of the list of your priorities. This may go against the grain, but it is not as selfish as it sounds. We can only cope positively with others when we can cope positively with ourselves. In an ideal world, this essential self-indulgence which helps us to get our priorities right means doing what we want when we want, but, as we all know, life is rarely that simple. Here are some things we can do.

★ Try to remove all unnecessary hassles from day-to-day life. For example, for as long as is necessary, see only those people you want to see. If you drive to work, would it be easier to use public transport a few days a week? Could you work from home some days? Could you lessen the frequency of any other stressful activities?

★ To give yourself breathing spaces, delegate, where possible, tasks that you need not do yourself, and try to organise your work and chores so they take up the minimum amount of time. List activities in order of priority and do the important things first. The less important things can wait.

★ Be realistic about what you can achieve and if you need help, and it is possible to get some, ask for it.

★ A problem shared is a problem halved. For example, if you cannot tell your boss about your work problems, share them with your partner, family, friends or workmates. Feeling stressed is nothing to be ashamed of.

★ Allow at least an hour of 'quality time' every day. Quality time is time spent doing what you want to do, what you enjoy doing and what makes you feel better. This can mean anything from sitting quietly reflecting, reading a book, going out for a drink with friends, or sitting down for a chat with your partner and family.

★ Indulge in a hobby – walking, gardening, bird watching, attending an evening class, swimming, theatre going, meeting like-minded people. All these are effective ways to switch off from the cares of the day.

★ Learn some relaxation techniques to ease away the stress. These are the basis of many stress management courses (see Relaxation therapies opposite).

Allow at least an hour of 'quality time' every day, doing what you want to do.

Relaxation therapies

It is very easy for someone who is stressed to dismiss relaxation therapy as a self-indulgent use of, or waste of, time. It will not, it is reasoned, pay the mortgage, reduce the pile of ironing or help meet crucial work deadlines. So, why bother?

The good positive effects of relaxation therapies, however, should never be underestimated or lightly dismissed. Whatever the stress, learning to relax will help you to feel better and more able to cope. Doctors certainly appreciate this and frequently recommend more and more variations of relaxation therapies.

Important and positive physiological changes take place during relaxation. These mirror – and counteract – the negative changes induced by stress in the first place. So, far from being a waste of time, learning to relax gives you a sound basis from which to tackle problems.

Breathing exercises: the most fundamental and time-honoured relaxation therapy is breathing exercises (see Breath of life, page 114). Breathing deeply is a powerful antidote to stress, and is the cornerstone of most deep relaxation techniques.

Breathing patterns are a powerful indicator of our state of mind. Just think how your breathing rate changes in the most nerve-racking moments of your favourite thriller. You breathe much faster and shallower than normal. Likewise, when you are stressed, your breathing pattern changes to fast shallow pants, even hyperventilation (over-breathing). How many times were you told as a child – or even more recently – to calm down and take a deep breath.

Complementary therapies: for stress, these include meditation, yoga, massage and aromatherapy. Ask your GP about these soothing, calming, relaxation techniques, or contact the organisations listed at the end of the chapter (see Useful addresses, page 116). Above all, do not be put off by any preconceived notions you may have about complementary therapies – they really do have a lot to offer.

Although the beauty of relaxation techniques is that they can all be practised alone in the privacy of your home, it is a good idea initially to get professional help to introduce you to what is on offer and set you off on the right track.

Breath of life

Five minutes spent practising the following breathing exercise, ideally outside or in front of an open window, wearing loose-fitting clothes, is a very good way to start. The aim is to create a deep slow breathing rhythm. If you feel stressed before going into a meeting or making a telephone call, just three rounds of the following will help you to collect yourself, relax and cope better:

▶ Lie or sit down – whichever you prefer – but make sure that your head, neck and spine are free from constrictions and aligned.

▶ Breathe in deeply and slowly, concentrating on expanding your chest and pushing out your stomach, so that your lungs are filled to maximum capacity.

▶ When you breathe out do the reverse – pull in your stomach and chest – so that you push out as much air as possible.

WHAT NOT TO DO!

★ Don't turn to comfort props, such as cigarettes and alcohol, to help you cope. They will not, and invariably they make matters worse. Likewise, don't seek solace in comfort-eating. All that will happen is that you will end up putting on weight and being potentially fat as well as stressed!

★ Don't miss out on regular exercise and 'quality time' because you do not believe there are enough hours in the day. This is the start of a vicious downward spiral. Living in misery is very demanding on time, so there is always time to change things for the better!

★ Sleeping tablets and tranquillisers just delay the moment when you will need to face up to the cause of the stress. They also cover up symptoms in the short term, and in the long term can cause more problems than they solve (see Chapter Six).

The crisis point

There is a lot of truth in the old adage that a problem shared is a problem halved. If you feel you are crumbling and falling to bits under the stress, then your first step is to reach out and tell someone. This can be a relative, a close friend or someone at work.

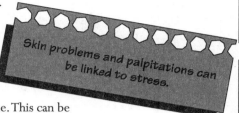

Skin problems and palpitations can be linked to stress.

If you feel you cannot share your problems with any of these people, then go to see your GP. Don't beat about the bush – no matter how silly or trivial you may fear your worries will seem to other people, they are obviously of paramount importance to you. Doctors do take such problems seriously and can often help patients to put things into perspective and work out a coping strategy.

Feeling suicidal?

If you are feeling really desperate and suicidal, with nobody to turn to, pick up the telephone and call the Samaritans. The number of the local branch will be in your telephone directory. The sooner you share your problem, the sooner you will discover that somebody cares and help is available. In such moments always keep in mind that many people who have attempted suicide have been very grateful later that they survived to live another day. We cannot know how those who succeeded would have felt if they survived, but, from the living proof of many survivors now working for the Samaritans, we can guess.

It is never too late to seek help, so, if you feel at the end of your tether, find the courage to reach out for help right now. It is there for the asking.

A healthy lifestyle is even more essential to someone who is stressed than somebody who is not.

GPs may not be able to provide all the solutions and can offer no quick fixes – we cannot prescribe holidays, a new job or help out with the mortgage or bills – but we can help people to find the solutions for themselves and offer them support while they do.

✉ Useful addresses

....

▶ Anti Bullying Campaign, 10 Borough High Street, London SE1 9QQ. Telephone: 0171 378 1446. Provides advice, information, understanding and support to parents of bullied children and to children themselves.

▶ Association of Physical and Natural Therapists, 93 Parkhurst Road, Horley, Surrey RH6 8EX. Telephone: 01293 775467. List available of registered practitioners and massage centres throughout the UK.

▶ British School of Yoga, The, 24 Hagley Road, Stourbridge, West Midlands DY8 1QD. Telephone: 01384 371320.

▶ British Wheel of Yoga, 1 Hamilton Place, Boston Road, Sleaford, Lincolnshire NG34 7ES. Telephone: 01529 306851. List available of registered practitioners and yoga centres throughout the UK.

▶ Institute for Complementary Medicine, PO Box 194, London SE16 1QZ. Telephone: 0171 237 5165 for a register of complementary therapists.

▶ International Federation of Aromatherapists, Stamford House, 2–4 Chiswick High Road, London W4 1TH. Telephone: 0181 742 2605.

▶ International Society of Professional Aromatherapists, 41 Ashby Road, Hinckley, Leicestershire LE10 1SN. Telephone: 01455 637987.

▶ Relate (formerly Marriage Guidance Council), Herbert Gray College, Little Church Street, Rugby, Warwickshire CV21 3AP. Telephone: 01788 573241. Offers help for couples with relationship difficulties.

▶ Royal College of Psychiatrists, The, 17 Belgrave Square, London SW1X 8PG. Telephone: 0171 235 2351. Self-help leaflets and factsheets on common mental health problems (including depression, anxiety and phobias, surviving adolescence). Send a stamped addressed envelope.

▶ Stress Busters, Personal Empowerment Programmes, 34 Denewood Avenue, Handsworth Wood, Birmingham B20 2AB. Telephone: 0121 551 2932.

▶ Transcendental Meditation, Freepost WN5 103F, Skelmersdale, Lancs WN8 6BR. Telephone: 0800 269303. Information pack and list of local classes available.

CHAPTER FIVE

'I'LL NEVER BE ABLE TO GIVE UP...'

★ Approximately 750 000 people stop smoking every year.

★ It is never too late to give up and reap health benefits from doing so.

★ If you really want to give up smoking, you will succeed.

★ If you do not want to give up, make changes to your diet and lifestyle which will substantially reduce the health risks.

WEDNESDAY'S CHOICE

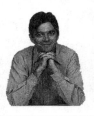

No Smoking

The first part of this chapter applies to everyone who smokes. It outlines the diseases and problems that are caused or made worse by smoking, and outlines the damage we do to our bodies every time we light up. Very worryingly, the latest research shows that the effects of smoking are even worse than doctors thought.

This information is important even if you are not yet interested in giving up. It is not all heart disease and lung cancer, and it might explain certain health problems you are experiencing right now. In time, it might even help you to want to stop smoking or at least cut down.

Personally, I believe that if people know about the health risks of smoking and still want to smoke, then that is their prerogative. But there is no excuse for ignorance, and every smoker should make sure they are fully aware of the health consequences both for themselves and those around them.

After the bad news, the rest of this chapter is divided into two sections – the first concentrates on ways to quit smoking; the second applies to people who do not want to give up, or simply believe they cannot at the moment. Tomorrow perhaps!

Sadly, I cannot offer any magic cures to help you give up – and neither can anyone else. So, don't believe all that you read or see advertised. Giving up can be hard but, take heart, 750 000 people manage to do it each year.

All too often doctors' attitudes to people who feel unable to give up is to tell them to change their mind or try harder! While quitting altogether is obviously by far the best option, I am aware that there are many facts that doctors do not take time to share with their patients, and some things that a 'hardened' smoker can do to help minimise the damage. Accepting that nearly a third of the population are continuing to smoke, and that some people are just not ready to give up, is not a dangerous or irresponsible stance for me, as a doctor, to take, it is simply realistic.

The really bad news

Tobacco smoke contains about 900 identifiable chemicals and over fifty of these are thought to be capable of causing cancer.

Although lung cancer was the first major disease to be reliably linked to smoking – and is still the disease mostly commonly associated with it – there are many other smoking-related diseases that actually have a higher death toll. In fact, cigarettes increase your chances of developing twenty-four fatal conditions: the top five are on the list.

★ Heart disease
★ Stroke
★ Cancer of the mouth, oesophagus, pharynx and larynx
★ Chronic pulmonary disease, such as emphysema and bronchitis
★ Osteoporosis

It is only recently that the true killing power of this weed has been fully appreciated. The researchers in Oxford who first identified the link with lung cancer in 1951 went on to follow up the subject with a group of doctors. The latest findings after studying smoking for a further forty years reveal:

▶ One in two regular smokers are eventually killed by the habit – with an average loss of sixteen years of life.
▶ The death rate among smokers in middle age is three times higher than that of non-smokers.
▶ In total, smoking-related diseases kill over twenty times more people each year than road accidents – 110 000 deaths a year in the UK alone.

It is not, however, just these major life-threatening problems – which often seem a lifetime away for smokers in their teenage years or twenties – that smokers should be aware of. Smoking has far-ranging and immediate effects on health.

Some of my patients get very defensive when I ask them about smoking. I can see them looking at me in a bored resigned way, thinking 'Yes, doctor, I do know what I'm doing to my lungs, thank you.' But many do not appreciate the effect their smoking is having on their health right there and then. Read on.

Sleeping problems: smokers are much more likely to experience these than non-smokers.

Infertility: smoking has a major effect on fertility, which is a growing problem today. Women smokers, for example, are three times more likely to take over a year to become pregnant than non-smokers; and male smokers often have a lower sperm count or less mobile sperm than non-smokers.

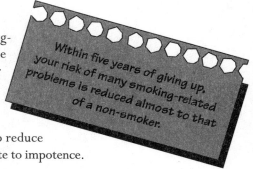

Within five years of giving up, your risk of many smoking-related problems is reduced almost to that of a non-smoker.

Impotence: smoking can also reduce the male sex drive and contribute to impotence.

Cervical cancer: women who smoke are four times more likely to develop cervical cancer.

Osteoporosis: smoking decreases bone density which greatly increases the risk of developing osteoporosis later in life. In women this risk is also raised in another way as smoking tends to bring the menopause on earlier, by an average of two years, which is itself a risk factor for osteoporosis.

Miscarriage: the risk of miscarriage is more than a quarter higher in smokers and smoking accounts for over 4000 miscarriages a year in England and Wales.

Premature labour: this is twice as common among smokers.

Stillbirths: the rate of stillbirths and early neonatal deaths is approximately one third higher – equivalent to about 420 deaths per year in England and Wales.

Low birth weight babies: babies born to mothers who smoke are on average 200 g (7 oz) lighter than babies born to non-smoking mothers.

Ageing: smoking ages skin tremendously, more so in women than in men as women's skin is thinner and so the damage is more obvious. The average thirty-five-year-old who regularly smokes twenty cigarettes a day can expect to have the complexion of a forty-five-year-old.

Nutritional deficiencies: smoking interferes with the way the body deals with certain nutrients – such as vitamin C, drugs and medications. For example the pain-killing effects of analgesics are reduced in smokers, who, as a result, often require higher doses.

Damage to blood vessels: most people are aware by now that smoking damages the walls of the arteries supplying the heart and that this leads to coronary heart disease. But perhaps it is not commonly known that smoking has a similar effect on blood vessels elsewhere in the body and those supplying the arms and legs are at particular risk.

Amputations: smoking is the biggest cause of amputations, which number over 2000 a year in England.

I could go on with the horrors but I guess you are getting the picture.

Smokers and the contraceptive pill

There are health risks associated with smoking and being on the combined contraceptive pill – and, ironically, women who take the pill are also more likely to smoke.

Oestrogen, one of the hormones in the pill, increases a woman's chances of a blood clot. In non-smokers this effect is negligible. However, add in smoking and these two factors combine so that the risk of blood clots is significantly raised, making the risk of a heart attack, stroke, or thrombosis, ten times more likely. As the total risk for the average twenty-year-old age group is still pretty small, I – along with most doctors – do prescribe the combined pill for these smokers, but I make sure they are aware of the risk. For women over the age of thirty-five, however, the risks start to get very much higher, and most doctors, including me, are not happy to prescribe the combined pill to smokers in this age range. Non-smokers on the other hand can continue to take the pill until their mid-forties.

Infants of parents who smoke are twice as likely to suffer respiratory illness.

WHAT'S IN A CIGARETTE?

Nicotine is the drug which makes smoking addictive. It is also a highly toxic chemical. It is important to remember that nicotine can be absorbed through your nose and mouth, so even if you are a member of the 'I don't inhale brigade', you can still get addicted.

Tar is made up of a number of carcinogens which contribute to respiratory disease and lung cancer.

Carbon monoxide interferes with the ability of blood to carry oxygen and can kill the delicate cells lining the blood vessels.

Young smokers

In 1992, about 10.6 million adults in England smoked cigarettes – about twenty-nine per cent of men and twenty-seven per cent of women. Figures from 1993 show that twenty-six per cent of fifteen-year-old girls and nineteen per cent of fifteen-year-old boys smoke regularly.

Research also shows that children who grow up with parents who smoke are three times as likely to smoke than children of non-smoking parents.

Passive smoking

The issue of passive smoking has taken centre stage recently in the smoking debate. The most extreme anti-smokers claim that they risk lung cancer every time they step into a pub. Pro-smoking supporters say that passive smoking is harmless and that the issue is primarily a propaganda device to make smoking a public evil rather than a private vice.

The controversy has now become so heated that it is hard to separate fact from fiction. To date, the only comprehensive research, from University College, London, on how much tobacco smoke non-smokers passively inhale reveals it to be the equivalent of one cigarette a week at most – and therefore one hundred times less of a health risk than the risks associated with other sources of air pollution. The Department of Health, however, estimates that about 300 non-smokers die each year from illnesses related to passive smoking.

The University College researchers concluded that passive smoking is an unlikely cause of lung cancer and I tend to agree with this. Passive smoking is unlikely to induce the major life-threatening diseases associated with smoking, but that is not to say that it has no effect on people's health. For example, there is little doubt that tobacco smoke can trigger asthma attacks in sufferers, and I certainly would not want an asthmatic patient working behind a smoke-filled bar in a pub.

What about the children?

There are many studies showing that smoking can affect the health of children. For example, infants of parents who smoke are twice as likely to suffer respiratory illness, and one-third of the cases of glue ear (a common cause of reversible deafness in young children resulting from the build up of sticky fluid in the ear after repeated ear infections) is attributable to parental smoking. Overall, it is estimated that approximately fifty children, under five, are admitted to hospital every day suffering from passive-smoking related illnesses.

The most serious and potentially fatal risk from passive smoking is to young babies. The latest research carried out by the Government's Confidential Inquiry into Stillbirths and Deaths in Infancy found that a baby whose mother and father smoke is five times more likely to die from Sudden Infant Death Syndrome (cot death) than a baby from a non-smoking home. If only the mother smokes, the risk reduces to three to four times more than that of non-smokers; and if only the father smokes, the risk is twice as high.

The tragedy of cot deaths leaves no room for any confusion about the need for parents of young babies to stop smoking.

Cutting down or switching brands

Reducing the number of cigarettes you smoke has massive health benefits and is certainly a major step to improving your health. The risk of virtually all tobacco related diseases goes up – and therefore down – in direct proportion to the number of cigarettes you smoke. I would rather see a patient cut down from twenty to five a day than try and give up for a few weeks, fail, and then go back to twenty a day.

I am less convinced about the supposed benefits of switching from high-tar cigarettes to low tar, because, in practice, smokers take longer and more frequent drags of low-tar cigarettes, thus defeating the objective. Having said that, as it is the tars in tobacco smoke that are linked to lung cancer and other respiratory diseases, in theory it should be a good move. It cannot hurt to try, but do not kid yourself you are taking a major step to lessening the risks and improving your health.

The benefits of giving up

Few hardened smokers cite health benefits as a major reason to stop smoking and this suggests that many think that the damage has already been done. Nothing could be further from the truth. There is absolutely no doubt that, however long you have smoked and however old you are, you will be healthier if you give up than if you carry on. In fact, giving up is, without doubt, the single most important thing anyone can do to improve their health.

The benefits on the heart and circulatory system are immediate. Blood is less likely to clot and the heart pumps more oxygen- and nutrient-rich blood around the body with less effort. Within five years of giving up, your risk of many smoking related problems is reduced almost to that of a non-smoker. Giving up after a heart attack can halve your risk of another heart attack virtually overnight. Ironically, it is much harder for a non-smoker actively to do something to reduce their chance of another heart attack.

After stopping smoking, the risk of stroke falls sharply in the first two years and, after five years, is about the same as that for a non-smoker.

It is not such good news for lung cancer because it takes about ten to fifteen years for this cancer to develop. So, in theory, you will still be at risk for this length of time after you stop smoking, but then the risk drops to pretty much the same level as that of a non-smoker.

In fact, the encouraging news is that studies show that men (there have been no studies yet on women) who give up under the age of thirty-five, on the whole do no worse in the long term than those who have never smoked.

GIVING UP

Psychological and physical factors: there are two sides to smoking – both of which need to be addressed if you want to turn your back on cigarettes once and for all. The one is the psychological dependence and the other is the physical dependence, or nicotine addiction.

Withdrawal symptoms: a lot is talked about nicotine addiction and the problems associated with withdrawal symptoms. Personally, I think this is blown out of proportion, although it is obviously wise to prepare yourself for it (see page 129). The withdrawal symptoms are a short-term problem and certainly do not explain why some people go back to smoking after several months or even years of abstinence.

The psychological factors are much more problematic. Smoking is an emotional crutch for many smokers, and people often tell me how smoking calms them or helps them cope with stress.

When you consider how difficult habits of any kind are to break, it is a wonder anyone ever succeeds in giving up smoking. Every time you smoke a cigarette you put your hand to your mouth at least ten times. If you are on twenty a day that is 200 times a day, 1400 times a week, 73 000 times a year – that is a big habit to break!

Wanting to stop: without a doubt, the most important factor in giving up is wanting to, and then putting the decision to do so into effect. Three-quarters of ex-smokers say their own willpower was the key to their success.

Making the decision to stop can take anything from days to years. But don't even try until you really and truly want to give up. Don't do it half-heartedly otherwise you will not succeed and simply become more and more convinced that you never will be able to kick the habit.

To want to give up, you have really got to sell the idea to yourself. Let me help you with the following reasons why you will be better off as a non-smoker.

Health reasons: I have already said that it is never too late to reap great benefits from stopping smoking. ▷

◁ **Social reasons:** smokers are already being made to feel like social lepers, banned from so many public places – and even relatives', friends' and colleagues' houses. If you want to see how much worse this anti-smoking situation is going to get, visit the United States where the reaction from the anti-smoking lobby is becoming ever more extreme.

Passive smoking: think about the people you live and work with – is it fair to expose them to your tobacco smoke?

Personal factors: think about prematurely wrinkled skin, yellowed teeth and fingernails, ashtray breath and stale-smelling hair, clothing and house – all caused by tobacco smoke.

Financial reasons: if you smoke twenty cigarettes a day you are spending over £20 a week and over £1000 a year on smoking. Think about how you could spend this money to reward yourself – a new wardrobe, a special holiday? It's all possible and up to you!

Motivators: Once you have decided to give up, write down all the reasons that have motivated you to do so and keep the list with you at all times. Read it when tempted!

Support network: I really cannot stress enough how important other people's support is to your success. Ideally, encourage your partner or a close friend, assuming one of them smokes, to give up at the same time as you. If not, and if it is unlikely that you will get support from your family or friends, then consult your GP. He or she will either offer their help or put you in touch with local support groups.

Tell people you do not smoke, not that you are trying to give up. As a non-smoker, you are far less likely to be tempted.

What about weight gain?

It is true that nicotine is an appetite suppressant and that cigarettes can act as a food substitute. So, yes, this can mean that smokers who give up can put on weight in the first few months.

The average amount gained is usually in the order of 1.75–2.25 kg (4–5 lb). But this is under your control. It is not the fact that you have stopped smoking that makes you put on weight, but the fact that you have substituted one comfort, smoking, for another comfort – eating! So, weight gain is not inevitable and you can take steps to avoid it.

Think up other non-comfort eating distractions. Start an exercise programme or a new interest (you can afford these now!) – anything that helps you to resist the temptation to turn to comfort eating to avoid the temptation of lighting up. Some people mention a craving for foods high in fat and sugar during the nicotine withdrawal period, so be prepared for this and make sure you have other less fattening foods available.

Finally, take heart from the fact that a smoking cessation expert told a group of medical students – including me – that each cigarette contains three calories!

Three steps to success

The key to success is really wanting to stop. In my experience, smokers who are pestered to quit by family, friends or doctors rarely succeed and simply remain convinced that they do not have the willpower.

Giving up is hard enough without starting in a half-hearted I'm-sure-to-fail manner. So, the first thing you have to do is convince yourself it is what you really want. Once you have made the decision, there are three stages.

★ Preparing to stop
★ Stopping
★ Staying stopped

Preparing to stop: choose a day to quit – it doesn't have to be New Year's Day or a national No Smoking Day – you don't have to run with the herd. Choose a time when you have the least number of tensions and other unhelpful distractions, and can focus on the resolution in hand.

Smoke twice as many as normal immediately before you quit – really overdo it, so that the smoke irritates your eyes and your throat – and until the thought of another cigarette makes you feel thoroughly sick.

Assess why, when and with whom, you are most at risk of smoking. Avoid, if possible, these situations and people for a while after you have stopped.

Do not empty your ashtrays – simply empty their contents into a glass jar, dampen the butts with a little water, and sniff this ghastly concoction before you smoke your last few cigarettes. After you have given up, get rid of all your smoking paraphernalia – ashtrays, lighters, etc.

Plan how to spend the money saved to reward yourself.

Stopping: Drink lots of water or fruit juice on the first day to help your body flush the toxins out of your system.

If you have a craving, select a substitute distraction – activity – that most fulfils the need that you think you smoked for.

If you need to put something in your mouth for substitute oral satisfaction purposes, make sure it is healthy and non-weight gaining – for example, sugar-free chewing gum.

If you need to do something with your hands, find something to fiddle with – a bean bag, worry beads – anything but a cigarette.

If you experience strong cravings and the need to smoke, try a displacement therapy, such as going for a walk, or relaxation exercises.

Tell people you do not smoke, not that you are trying to give up.

Staying stopped: always take it one day at a time – it is easier to think you will not smoke today rather than forever.

Take particular care after the first few weeks – do not become complacent and do not allow yourself to be tempted.

Think positively – always remembering and reminding yourself why you have stopped smoking.

Never use a crisis or celebration as an excuse for just one cigarette – there is no such thing.

If you do slip, then do not

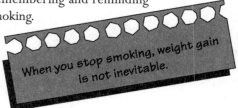

When you stop smoking, weight gain is not inevitable.

think this is the end of the world, that you are a worthless worm, total failure, and give in. Above all, do not use one failure as an excuse to start smoking again. Shrug it off. Walk on. Think of it as a minor set back and start again – the next time will be easier. Learn from your mistakes and do not make the same ones again. You will succeed in the end.

NICOTINE WITHDRAWAL

Nicotine is an addictive drug. It is a psychoactive substance that works at specific sites in the brain as a relaxant, and elsewhere as a stimulant. The US Surgeon General has compared tobacco addiction with that of heroin and cocaine, but the tobacco industry, for obvious reasons, only admits that it is habit forming – in the same realm as watching TV or drinking coffee!

You will have to be prepared for the physical effects of withdrawal, although the actual severity varies greatly from person to person. And, as I have stressed before, the psychological deprivation is harder to cope with than the physical.

Symptoms: the most common withdrawal symptoms are a decrease in heart rate and blood pressure, difficulty in sleeping, vivid dreams, and restlessness. Increased coughing is common as the functioning of the respiratory system improves and enthusiastically takes on the job of clearing out mucus and other junk from the lungs.

Dry mouth, slightly sore throat and, possibly, sore gums and tongue may also occur.

The psychological problems include distress, cravings, nervousness, tension, depression, irritability and fatigue.

The good news is that if you are determined and do not give in, these symptoms will probably only last a couple of weeks, while the benefits will last a lifetime. Look on the symptoms as positive signs that freedom is at hand, your body is recovering from the effects of tobacco, and you have actually given up nothing but health risks and potentially fatal diseases!

Nicotine replacement therapies

You might want to consider nicotine replacement therapies to ease nicotine withdrawal symptoms and enable you to tackle the psychological dependence or addiction first. These therapies deliver nicotine via a less hazardous means than smoke inhalation. They are available as chewing gums, skin patches and a nasal spray. But be warned: con artists have already jumped on the bandwagon and produced cut-price patches. Most of these are useless and should be avoided. Stick to branded, tried and tested names, available from your pharmacist who will be happy to advise you.

Do not, however, expect nicotine replacement therapy to be a miracle cure and do all the work for you. One study following up patch users a year after they stopped smoking showed that less than one in ten were still not smoking. This compared with one in twenty of placebo users – people who were given a 'dummy' patch without any nicotine in it.

Unfortunately, your GP will not be able to prescribe these replacement therapies on the NHS. The Department of Health seems to think that if you can afford to smoke, you can afford to pay for the therapy, and to be fair this only costs about the same as twenty cigarettes a day. Even so, I think the DoH is taking an extremely short-sighted view on this matter. You may find it cheaper to get a private prescription because then you will not have to pay VAT.

The patches come with manufacturers' guidelines that suggest you should not use them if you have angina, if you have had a recent stroke, or are pregnant or breastfeeding. They should also be used with caution by people who suffer from high blood pressure, circulation problems or diabetes. While this advice is certainly technically sound, these groups of people should not smoke either! There is no doubt in my mind that nicotine patches are a safer bet than the cigarettes they replace. If in doubt, consult your GP.

Do not be tempted to use nicotine replacement therapy to help you cut back. Using patches, gum or sprays and continuing to smoke may actually increase the amount of nicotine you are getting and make stopping altogether much harder. Do not con yourself – use these therapies in the way they were intended, or not at all.

Other aids for giving up

Dummy cigarettes are plastic ones you don't light up. They are harmless, but have never been proven to be effective.

Herbal cigarettes contain tar and carbon monoxide, so they are by no means a safe 'dummy' alternative to smoking tobacco.

Hypnosis and acupuncture are reported to work for some people, but I think it comes back to motivation – the fact that these people are seeking help and seeing somebody supportive could be the reason for the successes.

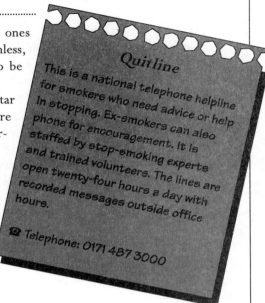

Quitline

This is a national telephone helpline for smokers who need advice or help in stopping. Ex-smokers can also phone for encouragement. It is staffed by stop-smoking experts and trained volunteers. The lines are open twenty-four hours a day with recorded messages outside office hours.

☎ Telephone: 0171 487 3000

How to be a healthier smoker

A healthy smoker may be a contradiction in terms; there are nevertheless some things that a smoker can do to reduce the risk.

Diet: one of the reasons that smokers' health is so bad is that so many of them are also renowned for taking little interest in, or care of, their own health. Characteristically, and compared to non-smokers, they eat much more meat and less fruit, vegetables and cereal, drink more alcohol and coffee, and are much more likely to be deficient in vitamins and minerals.

The Japanese have lower lung cancer rates than we do in spite of the fact that they tend to smoke stronger higher tar cigarettes. This is because their diet is much healthier than ours – lower in fat, higher in fibre, richer in antioxidant foods (see Chapter One), and the green tea they drink so much of is particularly protective. This is an unfermented tea containing chemicals, called flavonoids, which are antioxidants.

Smokers need to pay particular attention to what they eat and make sure they follow the guidance in Chapter One. When it comes to antioxidants it is true that tobacco smoke increases the amount of free radicals in your body (see Antioxidants and free radicals, page 34), but, as I explain in Chapter One, the case for taking megadoses of antioxidants is still far from proven. This makes it even more crucial for smokers to ensure that they eat about five to seven pieces of fruit a day. Many studies also show that smokers are deficient in vitamin C and, in this instance, I see no harm in smokers taking a supplement. Daily doses as high as 2000 mg are safe, but remember always to split the dose, taking half in the morning and half in the evening. I am also in favour of smokers taking vitamin E, as the evidence showing that this is cardio-protective is quite convincing. I am wary, however, at the moment of recommending smokers to take other vitamins and minerals for their antioxidant properties. (See Vitamins, Chapter One.)

Loss of calcium: smoking can lead to calcium loss, potentially weakening the bones, and, especially in women, can increase the risk of osteoporosis. The official recommendations are for 700 mg calcium a day, but some experts argue that higher levels are needed and that smokers should certainly strive for these. Dairy products are the best natural source of calcium, but remember they are also high in fat. If you think you are lacking calcium, you could consider a calcium supplement. Exercise is also important in keeping bones strong.

Cholesterol level: smoking, by damaging the lining of blood vessels, accelerates the pace at which fatty plaques build up in our arteries. I would certainly want smokers to establish their cholesterol level. If it is high, it means they need to pay particular attention to their diet, exercise and weight. (See Chapter One.)

High blood pressure: this is one of the most common health hazards of smoking, so make sure you get your blood pressure checked regularly by your GP. I would want to check my patients who smoke every three years at the very least. One of the best ways to lower blood pressure is through exercise. Regular exercise for six months can reduce blood pressure by about nine per cent. Smokers should also be particularly careful about watching their weight as this also raises blood pressure.

Exercise: studies have shown that smokers are generally far less active than their non-smoking peers. Like all people, smokers should do more exercise, and they have the added incentive that they will probably benefit from it even more than non-smokers. Smoking puts carbon monoxide into our bloodstream, thus reducing the amount of oxygen the blood can carry. A forty-cigarette-a-day person probably loses about seven per cent of their oxygen carrying capacity. This can be countered by aerobic exercise, which increases the lungs' ability to take up oxygen.

Exercise also helps lower cholesterol, blood pressure, and maintain a healthier body – all benefits that are additionally important in smokers who are already at risk of heart disease as a result of their habit.

Skin: in terms of premature ageing, smoking is one of the skin's worst enemies. A twenty-cigarette-a-day thirty-five-year-old can have the skin of someone ten years senior.

It is well established that smokers are more likely to have wrinkles than non-smokers. And there are a lot of different factors which cause this. Cigarette smoke contains chemical and pigments that can damage and stain the skin and destroy vitamin C which is essential for maintaining the structure of the skin. I always reckon on being able to spot a smoker in my consulting room just by looking at their skin! The older they are the easier this is.

Good basic skin care (see Chapter Three), avoiding the damaging effect of strong sunlight and taking vitamin C supplements, can help minimise some effects of smoking but not all.

In summary, it is never too late to give up. But remember the key to quitting is really wanting to do it in the first place. If you manage, and many people do, it is a decision you will never regret. If you do not want to give up, then do not despair; you can still take steps to minimise the harm you are doing to yourself. But please remember that there is no such thing as safe smoking – the only true way to be healthy is to become a non-smoker.

✉ Useful addresses

▶ ASH (Action on Smoking and Health), 109 Gloucester Place, London W1H 4EJ. Telephone:0171 935 3519.

▶ ASH Scotland, 8 Frederick Street, Edinburgh EH2 2HB. Telephone: 0131 225 4725. Helpline: 0131 226 5999.

▶ ASH in Wales, 372a Cowbridge Road East, Canton, Cardiff CF5 1HE. Telephone: 01222 641101.

▶ HEA Local Smoking Action Unit, University of the West of England, Oldbury Court Road, Fishponds, Bristol BS16 2JP. Telephone: 01179 762173.

▶ Quitline, Victory House, 170 Tottenham Court Road, London W1P 0HA. Telephone: 0171 487 3000 (for advice), 0171 388 5775 (for information).

▶ Ulster Cancer Foundation and ASH Norther Ireland, 40–2 Eglantine Avenue, Belfast BT9 6DX. Telephone: 01232 663281.

CHAPTER SIX

'I'D GIVE ANYTHING FOR A GOOD NIGHT'S SLEEP...'

★ Sleeplessness is never a problem in its own right — it is almost always a symptom of another condition or illness. Identify and treat this.

★ If you think a prescribed medication is keeping you awake, tell your doctor.

★ Nicotine, alcohol and caffeine are all sleep's enemies.

★ Do not make up lost sleep by catnapping throughout the day.

★ Don't work in your bedroom.

★ Sleeping tablets do not cure insomnia — they just cover up the cause and should be taken for short periods only.

★ Check your mattress is of the correct firmness and softness.

★ Snoring usually comes down to obesity, sleeping on your back or drinking alcohol.

THURSDAY'S CHOICE

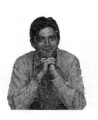

Sleep Better

Nothing beats a good night's sleep. I have to admit that I am exceptionally fond of mine, and am an eight-hour-a-night man. I do wish, though, that I was one of those fortunate people who get by on less. The only real problem I ever have with sleep is getting back to sleep after a disturbance. This means I dread night duty calls. Even when I get away with just one call at 2 a.m., I often lie awake for the rest of the night.

The occasional bad night's sleep, however, never hurt anyone. You may be a bit bleary eyed the next morning, but basically you just make up for the shortfall over the next few nights.

For many people, however, bed can become more of a battle zone than a refuge. One in four people experience some form of sleeping difficulty — from fitful sleeping to chronic insomnia.

Poor sleep does not just cause bad nights. I see patients who are quite literally at the end of their tether after weeks or even months of bad sleeping problems. The most common consequences are irritability, lack of energy and poor concentration. Spontaneity also falls by the wayside.

Lack of sleep can lead to underperformance and underachievement at work and in other activities, as well as being a major cause of accidents. As many as one in five motorway accidents, resulting in serious injury and death, are believed to be caused by sleepiness. Some drivers have even been spotted asleep behind the wheel in traffic jams or between lights changing from red to green.

Sleepiness has also been implicated in many of the world's major disasters – such as Chernobyl, *Exxon Valdez*, Bhopal and the *Challenger* space shuttle.

Sleep disturbances also have long-term effects. Some former shift-workers still suffer from high levels of sleep disruption ten years after adopting normal sleep patterns. And some researchers believe the high incidence of insomnia found in middle-aged and older women may be the result of disrupted sleep patterns during the baby and child-rearing phases of their life. Several studies have also shown that chronic insomnia is as powerful a predictor of early death as obesity.

Yet, historically, from a health point

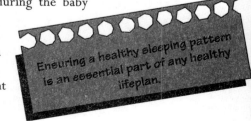

Ensuring a healthy sleeping pattern is an essential part of any healthy lifeplan.

of view, sleep disorders have been neglected and trivialised in the UK. In the USA and Canada, however, the opposite is true. They have had 'Wake Up' campaigns aimed at getting across the idea of just how important a good night's sleep is.

Fortunately, there is now a growing awareness of sleep problems in the UK, and many people who certainly would not have mentioned these to their doctor a few years ago are now coming in and asking for help.

This chapter, however, is not just for people who are experiencing sleep problems. It is important for everyone to appreciate the importance of sleep and understand a little about the causes of problems, so they can hopefully avoid them in the future. Ensuring a healthy sleeping pattern is an essential part of any healthy lifeplan.

SLEEP – THE FACTS

★ Most of us spend about twenty years of our life asleep.

★ Most adults need between six and eight hours' sleep a night, although there are exceptions, such as Margaret Thatcher, who was rumoured to get by on just three to four hours.

★ Newborn babies sleep for about sixteen hours a day, but wake often, drifting in and out of sleep during this period. As they get older they sleep for longer stretches, but for less time in total and the sleep becomes more concentrated during the night. By the age of three months nearly three-quarters are sleeping through until the morning.

★ The elderly sleep as little as six hours, although they often make up for this by napping during the day.

★ On average it takes about seven minutes to fall asleep.

Why do we sleep?

This is one of those awkward questions that doctors are often asked and find hard to answer. We know from studying patterns of brain activity that there are two distinct types of sleep – rapid eye movement (REM) sleep and non-REM sleep, also known as deep – or slow-wave sleep – which alternate throughout the night. REM sleep is the period when we dream and it is associated with marked physiological increases in temperature, heart rate, blood pressure and gastric acid secretion.

The most obvious and therefore most popular theory is that deep sleep is a period of recuperation – a chance for the body literally to recharge its batteries. Growth also occurs during this time. The periods of alternating REM sleep are thought to allow the body to get rid of waste products accumulated during these periods of recuperation.

This explains why when the need for sleep is greatest, for example, in babies, during pregnancy or after exercise, the amount of deep sleep increases along with the overall amount of sleep.

A second school of thought argues that this recharging effect is not so much needed for the body, but more importantly for the brain. Some doctors have suggested the presence of a mystery substance, substance S, which accumulates in the brain during the day and needs to be got rid of during the night. This may explain the association between psychiatric problems and a lack of sleep.

But even though we do not yet fully understand the true function of sleep, we appreciate from experience that it has restorative qualities, and is crucial to our health.

Insomnia

Experiencing difficulties with sleeping – insomnia – is surprisingly common, affecting about one in twenty people under the age of thirty and more than one in three pensioners.

It manifests itself in a number of ways: some sufferers cannot get to sleep in the first place, others constantly wake up throughout the night, or wake up very early in the morning and are unable to get back to sleep again.

Whatever the pattern, the frustration and disruption that insomnia causes are undeniable. Sometimes this problem only lasts for a short period of time and the cause, such as a major emotional disturbance, may be obvious. Chronic

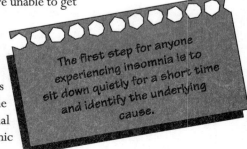

The first step for anyone experiencing insomnia is to sit down quietly for a short time and identify the underlying cause.

insomnia, however, can persist for weeks, months or even years, and some sufferers even resign themselves to it for the rest of their lives.

Traditionally chronic insomnia was treated as a disease in its own right and GPs simply prescribed sleeping tablets to anyone complaining about this problem. The medical profession now realises that this approach does more harm than good. In ninety-nine cases out of a hundred, there is a reason for the problem that needs to be investigated and the insomnia is simply an offshoot of this problem.

Programme yourself to turn off unpleasant thoughts and worries about the day.

The underlying cause can be a whole range of things – physical, mental or emotional in origin. For example, the pain associated with a physical illness, such as arthritis, can keep you awake; or you may be going through a ghastly divorce, or have lost your job. It could also be as simple as doing the wrong things before you go to bed.

The first step for anyone experiencing insomnia is to sit down quietly for a short time and identify the underlying cause. Doctors use a checklist which has become known as the Five Ps (see page 140).

It is a good idea to work through this list initially on your own, but if the cause is not obvious then ask your GP for help. Only when you know what it is that is causing the problem can you do something about it.

That aside, sleeplessness can become a problem in its own right. All too often people enter a vicious circle whereby they become so worked up about not sleeping that this makes it impossible for them to sleep. The scenario is common: you have had a spell of bad nights, so you become obsessed with getting a good night's sleep. You go to bed early, perhaps before you are tired, just to try and make sure you get those all important eight hours' sleep. Instead of sleeping, however, you spend most of the night tossing and turning, desperately trying to force yourself to sleep. The next night it is even worse, and so it goes on.

This vicious circle means that people can all too easily become trapped in an habitual pattern and the resulting problems persist long after the initial 'trigger' has ceased to affect you. Understanding how to break this vicious circle is very important (see Tackling insomnia, page 141).

THE FIVE Ps OF INSOMNIA

Physical: many physical illnesses prevent the onset of sleep or lead to arousals from sleep during the night. Most of us have been kept awake by a bad cough or cold but other illnesses, ranging from cardiovascular disease, tinnitus and pain, can all have the same effect. If you think that one of these, or any other physical problem, could be to blame, then ask your GP if he can help.

Physiological: getting to sleep is markedly affected by our activities immediately before bed. For example, late-night eating or stimulating exercise can keep you awake. Doctors have developed simple rules and routines which can help avoid such problems. This is called sleep hygiene and can be surprisingly effective (see page 142).

Psychiatric: anxiety, panic attacks, depression and mania all affect sleep and, in turn, the lack of sleep can make these conditions worse.

Psychological: worry – and stress – brought on by bad news or the thought of a difficult task the next day are common reasons for sleeplessness. I, for example, did not get a wink of sleep before my first appearance on morning television. These occasions only become a problem when the anxiety continues for any length of time. Just talking the problem over with close friends or family can help. If not, and if the problem is prolonged, your GP should be able to arrange counselling.

Pharmacological: many drugs interfere with normal sleep patterns. These include caffeine, alcohol, nicotine, beta-blockers, stimulants and some antidepressants. It is relatively easy to do something about the first three yourself (see page 141). But if you think that a prescribed drug is causing the problem, then ask your GP if there is an alternative drug you can use. Never, however, stop taking or reduce the recommended dose of a prescribed drug without first checking with your GP.

Tackling insomnia

Once the cause (or causes) of the problem has been identified, the next step is to tackle the problem. You may well need your GP's help, but I can well understand that if, for example, the cause is threatened redundancy and the loss of your job, you may feel the situation is hopeless and that no amount of advice from a doctor will help. In such an instance, it is most unlikely that a doctor's advice can dispel all your worries and concerns, but that is not to say that it is a waste of time. Book a session and try to follow some of the advice. (See also the self-help tips listed below).

Sleep's enemies

Although we rarely think of them as such, nicotine, alcohol and caffeine (in coffee and tea) are powerful drugs and have a marked impact on sleep problems. The solution lies in cutting down or stopping the intake. But do not expect the effects to be immediate, trials of abstinence may need to last several weeks before you appreciate the benefit.

Nicotine: although low blood concentrations of nicotine are known to have a mild sedative and relaxing effect, as the nicotine levels rise this effect is rapidly replaced by arousal and agitation. Smoking more than one cigarette within an hour of bedtime can delay the onset of sleep, while insomnia later on in the night can be caused by excessive smoking earlier on in the evening. Either way, the average smoker sleeps thirty minutes less a night than a non-smoker, and is certainly more likely to experience sleep disturbances.

The idea, however, that heavy smokers may have disturbed nights due to nicotine withdrawal and cravings for cigarettes in the early hours, is a common misconception. This fact has been confirmed by people who use twenty-four-hour nicotine patches. In reality, this treatment can occasionally cause even more sleep disturbance and, in addition, dreams and nightmares are a particular problem in some patients.

Alcohol: this is a sedative and it does help to promote sleep. However, before you decide this justifies more than one nightcap, think again because, although it helps to induce sleep, it diminishes the quality of sleep. During the night as the alcohol level drops the sedative effect wears off. As it approaches zero, there can then be a rebound effect which causes arousal – sweating, headaches and tachycardia (rapid pulse rate) – or intense dreams.

Caffeine: is a well-known pre-bedtime stimulant. But it is not just the caffeine you drink in the evening that affects sleep – it tends to hang around in the body a long time (up to six hours). An intake of 300 mg a day or more can certainly increase sleep problems, including the number of arousals from sleep. See the adjacent list for a guide to the caffeine content of drinks.

NB: other sources of caffeine include chocolate – 75 g/3 oz bar has a caffeine content of 40 mg; some drugs, such as Solpadeine, contain 30 mg per tablet/capsule; and Migril contains 100 mg per tablet.

Caffeine content (in mg) of drinks
(based on 150 ml/one average cup)

Roasted and ground coffee 80
Instant coffee 60
Decaffeinated coffee 3
Tea 30
Cola 15
Cocoa 20

Sleep hygiene

Sleep hygiene is the rather strange term that doctors use to describe the general advice they give concerning when, where and how people sleep. Although this advice is really aimed at people suffering from insomnia, to a certain extent it applies to all of us. I am not suggesting that you should never watch a film in bed or have a lie in – indeed I am very partial to both – but it is important for everyone to establish good sleeping patterns. Certainly it is worth sticking to the recommended guidelines opposite if you are experiencing sleeping problems.

Even though such measures sound simple, they have dramatically good effects on relieving sleeplessness. One American study showed that when the following tips became good behavioural habits, they cut the time a group of severe insomniacs spent awake by more than half, and they were much more effective than sleeping pills.

SLEEP HYGIENE

★ Avoid napping during the day. This can disrupt the pattern of night sleep.

★ Avoid strenuous exercise near bedtime. A gentle walk may help sleep, but anything more active should be restricted to earlier on in the day.

★ Only eat light snacks before bedtime and limit your fluid intake. Remember fatty foods take longer to digest and can cause indigestion or heartburn which will keep you awake.

★ Avoid substances such as caffeine, alcohol and nicotine close to bedtime.

★ Try to keep the bedroom temperature no higher than 18°C (65°F).

★ Don't work in your bedroom – reserve it for sleep and sex.

★ Go to bed only when you are sleepy-tired, rather than by convention or habit.

★ Put the light out immediately you retire. Don't watch TV in bed – this is an arousing activity.

★ If you don't fall asleep within twenty minutes of getting into bed, and are panicking or restless, get up, go to another room and do something relaxing until you are sleepy-tired.

★ Set the alarm for the same time every day and get up when it goes off.

★ Make sure your bed is comfortable and be prepared to buy a new one every ten years or so (see Buying a new bed, page 146).

Sleep disorders in children

Children, it must first be remembered, are individuals with individual needs. Some need more sleep than others, and some never seem to sleep for as long as we feel they should.

Sleep is a time of growth, so it is particularly important for children and adolescents. Likewise, although the need for sleep tends to lessen as children grow up, do not be too quick to judge adolescents as 'lazy'. The growth spurt around puberty means they really do need more sleep.

Sleep problems in children can have a devastating effect both on the child and the whole family, and sleep disturbances tend to fall into two categories – excess sleep or too little, interrupted sleep.

Excessive sleep: can be caused by a number of syndromes – one of which is sleep apnoea (see Sleep apnoea, page 153). In children this is usually caused by excessive tonsillar and adenoidal tissue and is easy to spot by the way in which these children sleep – usually on their elbows and knees with their bottom in the air. In most instances, as the children get older, the adenoids and tonsils start to shrink. If they do not, surgery might be the only option, and this is usually one hundred per cent effective.

Too little, interrupted sleep: the most common physical reasons for these in childhood are illnesses, such as asthma or eczema. I have seen the lives of whole families disrupted by these problems. The best thing to do in this situation is to make sure that the child is taking sufficient medicinal drugs to control the symptoms.

Interrupted sleep can also be caused by nightmares, night terrors or sleepwalking.

Nightmares are not uncommon and are often related to frightening films or viewing inappropriate television programmes. Unless the nightmares are really frequent, loving reassurance is probably all that is needed.

Night terrors are when the child does not wake, but stares into space often muttering. Usually the child has no recollection of this when waking up the next morning, and they are probably more frightening occurrences for Mum and Dad than for the child. They are more common in boys and tend to run in families. Although they usually occur during times of stress, they are not, in isolation, indicative of emotional disturbance, and children usually grow out of them.

Sleepwalking is quite rare. The major concern here is to make sure that doors and windows are secured so that the sleepwalker is unlikely to come to harm.

Anxiety and panic attacks: many children go through phases when they become anxious that their parents may disappear during the night – sometimes, for example, after a death in the family. These children may have trouble going to sleep or wake often during the night.

Bedtime routines: establishing a good bedtime routine that makes going to bed a happy pleasurable experience helps to overcome many problems.

This should include keeping an eye on pre-bedtime activities and ensuring they are not too exciting, over-stimulating or generating hyperactivity. Going to bed at a fixed time and reasonable hour, preceded by calming activities such as a bath and a bedtime story, are also a great help.

Sleepwalking is quite rare.

Battleground: be careful not to give into protestations after a prolonged battle about bedtime. This will merely serve to make a battle all the more likely the next night. Also make sure you do not reward wakefulness and calling out with long chats, stories, cuddles, etc. Try to get the balance right by giving enough comfort to reassure the child, but not so much that it encourages repeat behaviour. Give due praise and treats when your child sleeps through the night – and even make a record chart of when this happens and plan appropriate rewards.

The above suggestions are quite hard to put into practice, but when you do manage it they are pretty effective. Your GP will be able to give you more specific help, but there is very seldom a case for sleep-inducing drugs for children.

Sleep and the elderly

Sleep problems are more common in this age group and studies show that around fifty per cent of men and women over sixty experience them. The problem is exacerbated by catnapping during the day and not feeling tired at bedtime.

Likewise, the problem is made worse because many elderly people rely on hypnotics – sleeping pills which, up until the 1980s, doctors used to dole out for long periods before their potential to cause addiction was realised. Elderly users, however, often remain convinced of their value, even though the drugs are now known to be ineffective when taken for long periods.

Getting off to sleep is rarely a problem in the elderly, the more common problem is frequent awakenings during the night and/or waking very early in the morning.

Many factors can play a role, and it is always a good idea to see your GP. Identifying the cause of the problem can, for example, often lead to diagnosing an underlying physical or mental illness. Physical causes may be angina or palpitations, peptic ulcers, respiratory problems, or pain caused by diseases such as osteoporosis or arthritis.

Depression and dementia, very often ignored in the elderly, are also very strongly related to insomnia. One survey found that only one in five elderly depressed people were receiving a suitable medication – the rest just got a sleeping tablet. This record is appalling. Appropriate treatment of the true cause of insomnia is essential in elderly people, and will lead to improvements in daytime alertness and quality of life. So, if you are elderly and suffering from sleeplessness, don't accept insomnia as a natural consequence of ageing.

Buying a new bed

The National Bed Federation says a bed lasts an average of about ten years – although this obviously depends on the amount of wear and tear it gets and what quality the bed was in the first place. Although prices vary tremendously, the Federation recommends that, as a general guide, a good-quality bed will cost between £500 and £800 and give service for about ten years.

There is no doubt that a new bed can improve quality of sleep. One French study found that when chronic poor sleepers swapped their old bed for a new one, they got to sleep more quickly, woke up less frequently during the night and gained nearly an hour's extra sleep overall.

To make sure you have the right combination of comfort and support for you and your partner, always lie on the bed in the showroom before making your choice.

People with back problems are usually advised to check their mattress and to change, if necessary, to a firm or orthopaedic mattress. As there is, however, no set standard for these beds, be warned because the quality can vary quite tremendously.

Don't work in your bedroom – reserve it for sleep and sex.

A mattress that gives the right amount of support will hold your spine level. If the mattress is too soft, your body will sink into the mattress, affecting the alignment of the spine. If it is too hard, the mattress will not let the shoulders and hips sink in, but it will put uncomfortable pressure on other parts of the body.

Because it is essential to get this right, always, however daft you feel in the showroom, lie on your back on the bed and try to slip the palm of your hand between the mattress and the hollow of your back. If you can do this easily, the mattress is probably too hard for you; if it is very difficult, the mattress is probably too soft. Keep trying until you find the right one.

It is not just comfort that improves when we buy a new mattress – but hygiene, too. For example, we lose up to 500 g (1 lb) of skin a year and most of this (sorry, charming thought) makes its way into the bed.

Currently, the most popular bed size in the UK is the narrowest and shortest in the world – 135 x 190 cm (4ft 6in x 6ft) – so the chances are that, in the beds throughout our land, a lot of people's feet are dangling over the end of the bed. In more sensible countries, such as Belgium, Greece, Holland and Switzerland, people favour bigger beds – usually 160 x 200 cm (5ft 3in x 6ft 5in).

Ideally a bed should be at least 15 cm (6 in) longer than the tallest person using it.

House dust mites

These microscopic creatures share our homes, living in soft furnishings, particularly our beds. They, or rather the dung pellets they produce, are one of the commonest causes of allergies, such as asthma, eczema and rhinitis (an itchy, runny nose). Old mattresses and bedding are recognised as the chief source of contact with the asthma allergen found in the faecal pellets of house dust mites. Washing bedding at temperatures of 55°C (130°F) kills dust mites, and regularly vacuuming the mattress also helps. Mattress barrier covers are now available and are particularly recommended for asthma sufferers.

Airing the bed every day helps to control the dust mite population, as well as allowing the 600 ml (l pint) or so of body moisture that we lose every night to evaporate.

The National Asthma Campaign has produced a leaflet on house dust mites, which can be obtained by sending a large stamped addressed envelope to the address at the end of this chapter.

The mites thrive in warm, damp, dusty conditions and live off human skin scales. As we all shed up to one gram a day, they are rarely hungry. Although they have no adverse effects on most people, they do 'trigger' allergic reactions in others. Studies show that if people with asthma move into environments that are free from dust mites, their symptoms improve.

Having said that, it is quite difficult to reduce the number of dust mites in the home without getting rid of carpets, curtains and family pets! Taking the following points into consideration is more realistic and will help:

▶ Air the bedroom every day.
▶ Wash bedding, including pillows and duvets, regularly.
▶ Washing temperatures of above 55°C (130°F) kill dust mites.
▶ Vacuum all rooms vigorously, paying particular attention to the sides of fitted carpets and corners, behind and under beds and other furniture.
▶ Once a week, include your mattress and soft furnishings in the vacuuming routine.

Remember there is not much point in vacuuming if you are using a vacuum cleaner that recirculates the dust you collect back into the air. Unfortunately, this is what happens with many standard cleaners, including the so-called high efficiency versions. Opt for a vacuum cleaner containing fine filters which prevent the re-emission of dust particles. Many modern vacuum cleaners now come with these as standard.

★ Wash teddy bears and other soft toys or put them in the freezer to kill dust mites.
★ Exclude all pets from bedrooms.
★ Replace old bedding.
★ Buy covers which are impermeable to dust mites for pillows and mattresses.
★ Place air-filters or ionisers in bedrooms.
★ Consider using chemical sprays (available from chemists) to keep the number of dust mites down or neutralise the allergen in their droppings.

Relax!

Relaxation is often the key to a good night's sleep – particularly if you are becoming trapped in the vicious circle I mentioned earlier. Working yourself up into a frenzy is the very worst thing you can do. There are lots of different ways to relax and how we choose to do this depends on individual preferences. The following ideas may be helpful.

Biofeedback exercises are becoming increasingly popular. The idea here is that stress and anxiety produce subtle changes in the skin which can be detected by using a device that measures the electrical resistance of the skin. A range of these machines are available from pharmacists and medical suppliers. The most common type uses either a high pitched tone or a series of clicks. The more relaxed you are the lower the tone and the less frequent the clicks. By using these machines, plus a variety of relaxation techniques, it is possible to learn how to relax effectively.

Other ways to relax include deep breathing, muscle stretches or yoga exercises (see Chapter Four).

Programme yourself to turn off unpleasant thoughts and worries about the day that has just been or the one just coming. A common problem is that bedtime is often the first chance some people have to look back over the day or think about the next one which, of course, overstimulates the mind just when you need to relax. If this is a problem it is a good idea to set aside twenty minutes early on in the evening to reflect on all the things you normally start worrying about in bed.

SOME GOOD RELAXATION TIPS

★ Never try to fall asleep. The effort will keep you awake!

★ Tell yourself sleep will come when it is ready and that relaxing in bed is the next best thing.

★ Keep your eyes opened in the darkened room until you really cannot stop them closing.

★ Visualise a pleasant landscape or repeat a neutral soothing word every few seconds.

Always bear in mind that you may be expecting too much from a night's sleep. Yes, sleep is restorative, but do not expect miracles. It cannot make up for a basic lack of balance in your life, especially if most of your days are hectic. It may well be more constructive to concentrate on changes to your daytime rather than to your night-time routine.

COMPLEMENTARY THERAPIES

These have a good record when it comes to insomnia and many people claim they can help us to relax before bedtime. There are many books devoted to this subject (see Further reading on page 173).

Massage: treat yourself or ask someone to give you a soothing relaxing massage before you hit the sack. If nobody is available, try self-massage (included in most good massage books – see Further reading on page 173) of the feet and face. This can be as effective, if not as much fun!

Herbal remedies: everyone I know recommends a cup of camomile tea as a good way to encourage sleep. The herb valerian is also effective – about twenty drops in water half an hour before bed. Lavender oil may also help – some hospitals regularly vaporise this oil or put it on patients' pillows to induce better sleep.

Yoga: is another form of complementary medicine that has proved popular as a treatment for insomnia. It is basically a form of relaxation combined with meditation. Twenty minutes a day will help to improve mobility and flexibility as well as to reduce stress and tension. It is a good form of gentle exercise for older people.

Medication

The first option for many people who favour the medication route is a quick trip to the chemist, and in recent years a number of over-the-counter preparations have become available.

Diphenhydramine: the latest sleep-inducing offerings contain a drug called diphenhydramine which is an old-fashioned antihistamine which, like many other antihistamines (for example, Piriton) has marked sedative side-effects.

Diphenhydramine can also be found in a number of night-time cold and flu remedies. Its use as a sleeping aid, however, is controversial. Apart from its side-effects, my main worry is its duration of action. People taking diphenhydramine at night still have the drug in their system thirty-six hours later – thirty hours longer than they need it. Far from feeling refreshed the next morning, some people feel muzzy and tired, the very feeling they were trying to avoid in the first place.

Sleeping tablets: hypnotics or sleeping tablets, of which the benzodi-azepines (the Valium family, for example, temazepam and Mogadon) are probably the best known, are among the most commonly prescribed drugs in the UK with about fifteen million prescriptions being written each year.

Most of this is a hangover from the time when GPs simply doled out sleeping tablets to anyone complaining of insomnia. We now know, unfortunately to our patients' cost, that this remedy has caused more problems than it has solved. Firstly the body develops a tolerance to these drugs, which means they simply stop working after a relatively short period of time. More worrying is the fact that they are potentially addictive. Even short courses of a few weeks can lead to problems. Many patients find that when they stop taking the drugs they cannot sleep (rebound insomnia). This normally settles down after a few days, but, in the meantime, the problem may encourage people to continue taking the drug for long enough to become addicted to it.

The benzodiazepines act in a similar way to alcohol and can make patients very wobbly and prone to falling over if they get up in the night, or even in the case of the longer-acting types (for example, Nitrazepam) the next day. This is particularly dangerous in elderly people who are at high risk of bone fractures.

Hypnotics really only have a place in the treatment of transient insom-nia, for example caused by jet lag or acute stress during a divorce or after a bereavement. If they are used in these circumstances, they should be used only as a brief stop-gap measure while the true underlying problem is dealt with. I prescribe temazepam or Zopiclone for short courses of ten days to two weeks.

Snoring

....

Losing weight can be a surprisingly effective way to deal with snoring.

This affects about one in five middle-aged people and becomes more common with increasing age. Traditionally, snorers are the butt of many a joke but doctors now take the condition seriously and offer help.

The characteristic sound of snoring is caused by vibration of the soft palate and uvula. The soft palate is the fleshy part at the back of the roof of the mouth and the uvula is the 'dangley thing' that hangs down from it (the part most people erroneously think is their tonsils).

Although I always, as a matter of course, examine someone for physical deformities, snoring usually comes down to one or more of three things – obesity, sleeping on your back and drinking alcohol.

Losing weight can be a surprisingly effective way to deal with snoring. Just losing 6.5 kg (1 stone) can do the trick, and bear in mind you do not have to be very overweight for this to be a factor.

The best way to avoid sleeping on your back is to sew a pocket into the back of your pyjama top and put a golf ball in it or some other small object. Or, as Dame Edna Everage once told me, put two tennis balls in an old bra and put it on back to front! Simple but effective.

Alcohol leads to snoring because it relaxes the muscles in the nose and throat. It is dose related – I would not expect anyone to snore after just one glass of wine, but ten pints of beer is a different matter!

Because snoring is such a common problem, there are many devices on the market which claim to help. My favourite is a device that straps to your wrist, picks up the sound of snoring and gives you an electric shock. I am not sure that it helps very much, but it certainly gives your partner a lot of satisfaction!

Others include tubes that stop your nostrils collapsing and a tongue-retaining device that looks like an inverted dummy. Although it is easy to laugh about these gimmicks, some people are prepared to try anything to stop snoring – even surgery, which is available on the NHS. Surgeons use a laser to burn a straight line on the back of the soft palate which, having scarred, then stiffens the palate and makes it less likely to flap. This procedure only takes about fifteen minutes and is performed under local anaesthetic.

I would not recommend surgery for someone who just snores a bit on Saturday night after a few pints, but it is certainly a very quick and useful solution for patients with more severe snoring problems.

Last but not least, it is important to remember that there are two patients – the snorer who is often blissfully unaware of the problem and his or her partner, the 'snoree', who is invariably the one who makes the appointment with the doctor. Both need to be treated with sympathy. I have learned over the years never to underestimate the friction that can exist between the two parties – I even had one patient who asked me if she could use snoring as grounds for divorce! (See also Sleep apnoea, below).

Sleep apnoea

Snoring is linked to a condition called sleep apnoea, where the snorer stops breathing for periods of between seconds and a couple of minutes. This occurs when the upper airway at the back of the throat is sucked closed when the person breathes.

The resulting struggle to breathe usually wakes the person, albeit very briefly. This can happen up to 1000 times a night, although, in contrast to their long-suffering bed partner, the sufferer is often totally unaware of it. However he or she will be aware of severe fatigue the next day and sleepiness – even though they think they have had a good night's sleep.

Sleep apnoea, which is usually diagnosed from the partner's descriptions or by monitoring the patient in a sleep laboratory, is recognised as a major cause of ill health and is linked to an increased risk of heart attack and strokes. The Royal College of Physicians estimates that it is responsible for 700 deaths a year.

One effective treatment is to use a continuous airway pressure mask. The patient has to wear a mask connected to a fan unit which acts like a pneumatic splint by keeping a continuous flow of air moving through the airways. The snorer needs to breathe out against the air flow, which means that the pressure of the system has to be very carefully adjusted.

Circadian rhythms

Tiredness is not just related to how long we have been awake. Our bodies are controlled by internal biological clocks kept in time by exposure to daylight. Light falling on the back of the eye inhibits the production of a hormone in the brain called melatonin, the hormone recently hailed as the latest anti-ageing miracle drug. Although I would be wary of these claims, it has been used to counter the effects of jetleg and improve sleep patterns successfully. High levels of melatonin occur during the night with the lowest levels occurring just after midday. High levels of melatonin induce drowsiness. This means any breaks from our normal routine are harder to cope with, particularly if much of our time is spent indoors or working in an artificially lit environment. This particularly applies to shift workers and frequent air travellers (see Jet lag, below).

Researchers in America have been helping people with long-term sleep problems to reset their biological clocks by exposing them to bright lights that simulate daylight first thing in the morning and getting them to wear sunglasses in the evening.

Light, however, is only one factor that controls our alertness throughout the day. Levels of hormones in our blood vary and this is one reason why many of us notice that we are at our best in the morning and early evening but tired in the early afternoon and late at night. This early afternoon tiredness explains the popularity of the siesta, particularly in hot climates. But be warned, sleeping during the day will decrease the amount of sleep you need at night and often makes insomnia worse.

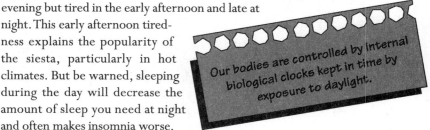

Our bodies are controlled by internal biological clocks kept in time by exposure to daylight.

Jet lag

This is a common problem for people crossing several time zones, particularly if they are travelling east to a country where the time difference is more than five hours. Symptoms may include headache, appetite loss, irregularities in bowel movements, poor concentration, sleepiness during the day and sleeplessness at night – the sort of symptoms that can ruin the first few days of a holiday or decrease a businessman's effectiveness at that all-important board meeting. .

These symptoms usually decline after a few days because, generally speaking, our body clock then falls in line with the time cues of the new environment. Ironically, jet lag probably affects business men who spend their time in constant meetings more than holiday-makers. This is because the former are not exposed to natural sunlight which is probably crucial in realigning the internal clock.

When travelling, I make sure I set my watch as soon as I board the plane to synchronise with my destination. I then live at the new timescale in terms of eating and sleeping patterns, both on the plane and when I arrive.

Always try to remain awake until your new bedtime, and if you are not tired rest in a darkened room. Avoid naps as these will simply confuse your body all the more.

Jet lag is one instance when sleeping tablets can be particularly effective – although doctors differ on whether this is appropriate use of NHS resources.

SHIFT WORK

The effects of shift work are similar to those of jet lag, but obviously it affects people for longer periods of time. Chronic fatigue and sleep problems are often a major reason for people leaving shift work, assuming they have a choice. The following points will help:

★ Nap before going to work at night.
★ Try and get shifts rotating clockwise – morning, daytime evening, night-time, etc.
★ Have, if possible, a slow rotation of shifts.
★ Before starting a night shift, go to bed progressively later.
★ Improved physical fitness can combat sleepiness during the night.
★ Try to avoid exposure to bright light in the morning when in bed.

✉ Useful addresses

▶ British Acupuncture Council, Park House, 206 Latimer Road, London W10 6RE. Telephone: 0181 964 0222.

▶ British Society of Hypnotherapists, 37 Orbain Road, London SW6 7JZ. Telephone: 0171 385 1166.

▶ Medical Advisory Service, PO Box 3087, London W4. Telephone: 0181 994 9874.

▶ National Asthma Campaign, Providence House, Providence Place, London N1 0NT. Telephone: 0171 226 2260; helpline: 0345 010203.

▶ National Bed Federation, The, 251 Brompton Road, London SW3 2EZ. Telephone: 0171 589 4888.

▶ National Institute of Medical Herbalists, 56 Long Brook Street, Exeter, Devon EX4 6AH. Telephone: 01392 426022.

CHAPTER SEVEN

'CHEERS! FANCY ANOTHER?'

★ Three units of alcohol increases happiness but significantly impairs judgment.

★ Anyone whose health is affected by alcohol – whether physically, emotionally, socially or psychologically – is a problem drinker.

★ Women's bodies are more affected by alcohol than men's.

★ It takes one hour for your body to remove each unit of alcohol from your bloodstream.

★ Alcohol reaches the brain within five minutes of being swallowed.

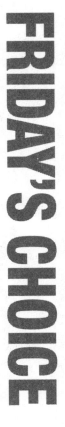

FRIDAY'S CHOICE

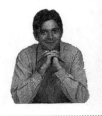

Drink Wisdom

CHANGES THAT COME ABOUT WITH INCREASED BLOOD LEVELS OF ALCOHOL

Pub unit measures: 1 unit = ½ pt beer; glass of wine; single spirit measure.

Units of alcohol	Effect on a normal-weight man
Up to two	Cheerfulness and increase in self-confidence.
Two	Increased risk of having an accident.
Three	Usually increased happiness, but significantly impaired judgement.
Five	Above legal limit for driving. Potential loss of driving licence and cause of serious and fatal accidents to self and others.
Ten	Slurred speech, loss of self-control.
Twelve	Inability to walk straight and loss of memory.
Eighteen	Approaching toxic levels. Continued drinking will be dangerous and may lead to unconsciousness.

Drinking copious amounts of coffee, enduring a cold shower or taking a walk in the fresh air will not make the slightest difference to counteract the effects of a heavy drinking session.

However much we may enjoy a drink, alcohol has always been regarded by doctors as bad news or, in the words of the Royal College of Physicians in 1726, and more recently in 1991, as a 'great and growing evil'. A few years ago the British Medical Association (BMA) even forced its wine society underground – not that this stopped doctors drinking. Unfortunately doctors are often better at giving advice than taking it, and are among the heaviest drinkers in the country. As a result, some people may call doctors hypocrites, but I think it is simply that, whatever their personal weaknesses, doctors want the best for their patients.

The good news for people who enjoy an occasional drink is that recent studies, involving hundreds of thousands of people, have shown that moderate alcohol consumption protects us against heart disease, and is actually better for us in this respect than abstention. Much of this research has centred on red wine, which may contain additional protective factors, but most forms of alcohol are now thought to share this good effect.

It is an interesting finding and one that helps to explain why the French, the biggest drinkers in Europe, seem to have such a low incidence of heart disease despite the fact that they smoke more and exercise less than we do. This statistical anomaly is known as the French Paradox.

This reassuring evidence, however, is still somewhat controversial. The problem is that many doctors do not like this message because they regard the idea that alcohol may be good for us as dangerous information. And there is good reason for their caution. Alcohol contributes to 25 000 deaths a year and, after cancer and heart disease, is the third major health hazard in this country. One in four medical hospital beds are occupied by patients with alcohol-related conditions.

As always, it is a matter of striking the right balance. So, while not preaching abstinence, I do think it important that everyone understands the effects that alcohol can have on our health. Only then are we able to make an informed choice about what is appropriate for ourselves.

Blood alcohol level increases with every unit you drink (see table opposite). But, while intake can rise rapidly, getting it out of the system is another matter.

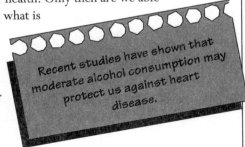

Recent studies have shown that moderate alcohol consumption may protect us against heart disease.

MEASURING ALCOHOL INTAKE

First the basics. To understand the amounts of alcohol referred to and to work out your own weekly intake, you have to know what makes up a unit of alcohol. Unfortunately alcoholic drinks are not labelled with the number of units they contain. Use the following guidelines to calculate your weekly intake.

One unit is equivalent to 10 ml (2 teaspoonsful) of pure alcohol and is found, for example, in half a pint of ordinary strength lager or beer, a glass of wine or a single measure of spirits. Do not forget these are pub measures not the measure you might help yourself to at home. And do watch out for strong lagers and beers.

The current sensible limits are twenty-eight units a week for men and twenty-one for women.

Alcohol is removed from the bloodstream and broken down by the liver. But the liver is like a car with only one gear and, on average, we can only burn one unit an hour, although this is increased in heavy drinkers.

So, if you have drunk four pints of beer (eight units) it will take eight hours before your blood alcohol level is back to zero. This obviously has very important — and dangerous — implications for the morning after, and a person who has drunk heavily the night before may still be over the legal limit when driving to work the next day.

Contrary to popular belief, drinking copious amounts of coffee, enduring a cold shower, or taking a walk in the fresh air will not make the slightest bit of difference to counteracting the effects of a heavy drinking session.

How much do we drink? In 1993, the average person over fifteen years drank 247 pints of beer or lager, and nearly 4 litres (7 pints) of pure alcohol in the form of wine and spirits. This figure was fifty per cent up on the average consumption in 1963.

How alcohol affects us

Alcohol is absorbed through the walls of the stomach and small intestine from where it enters the bloodstream. It starts to reach the brain within five minutes of being swallowed. Contrary to popular thinking, it is a depressant rather than a stimulant and subdues brain activity.

Its effect on the brain itself – and behaviour – reflects the way the brain is organised. It interferes with the function of the most advanced parts of the brain first and then, as more is drunk, it affects the lower brain systems.

The first parts to be affected are the frontal lobes of the brain responsible for co-ordinating plans and actions. They are also the seat of self-awareness, forethought and impulse control – the very faculties that are most vulnerable to a few drinks. As this part of the brain is effectively in charge, when its function is impaired the lower levels also begin to malfunction as they are released from its control. The next to suffer is the cerebral cortex which controls complex reasoning, calculation, language, memory and perception. Hence the slurring of speech and loss of reason that accompanies too much drink.

Next down the brain hierarchy are the parts which control memory, emotion, hunger, thirst and libido (sex drive). Further down still are the parts of the brain responsible for basic alertness, breathing, heart rate and co-ordination of movement. This is why continued drinking leads to swaying and staggering, increasing drowsiness and even unconsciousness.

The chart on page 158, Changes that come about with increased blood levels of alcohol, shows the approximate amounts of alcohol that bring about these changes. In practice, however, do remember that there is massive individual variation depending on how quickly the alcohol is drunk, the amount of food that has been eaten (food slows down the absorption of alcohol), and a person's degree of tolerance, which varies greatly from one individual to another.

Women and alcohol

The following is not a sexist comment. Drink for drink, most women will end up with a higher blood concentration of alcohol than men. A general rule is that a woman who drinks two glasses of wine will have a similar blood alcohol concentration to a man who has had three glasses.

There are two physiological reasons for this. Firstly, alcohol is distributed throughout the body's fluids and men have proportionately more of these (sixty-five per cent of a man's body weight is water compared to only

HANGOVERS

Most of us have been plagued with a hangover at some time. And we all have our own cures. These are the main symptoms and causes of hangovers.

★ Feeling shaky, nauseous and clammy is often a direct result of falling blood alcohol levels and these are the classical signs of alcohol withdrawal. In very heavy drinkers this can be compounded by a low blood sugar (hypoglycaemia) which causes similar symptoms.

★ The headache, dry mouth and raging thirst are caused by dehydration. Alcohol is a diuretic which means it makes the body get rid of water – that's why you often need to go to the loo after a few drinks.

★ Headaches can also be caused by congeners, a group of substances which are formed during the fermentation of dark coloured drinks such as red wine, brandy and port. Most people have noticed that they get a worse hangover after drinking red wine or brandy than from white wine or vodka – unit for unit that is.

★ Alcohol is an irritant and heavy drinking can lead to inflam-mation of the stomach (gastritis) causing nausea and heartburn.

Increased tolerance to drink creates the need to drink more to have the same effect.

fifty-five per cent in women). This means that drink for drink and weight for weight, alcohol is more diluted in a man's body than in a woman's. Secondly, it also appears that men break down more alcohol in their stomach before it gets a chance to enter their bloodstream.

This is why the current sensible drinking limits differentiate between men and women. It also has repercussions for safe drinking limits – women should drink no more than two units if they intend to drive.

Hangover cures

Working on the above causes and symptoms it is easy to see what you need to do to cure a hangover. Unfortunately, in practice, it is not that simple. Some of the best known hangover cures, however, do have a scientific basis – albeit a shaky one.

▶ 'Hair of the dog.' This expression originates from the old belief that taking a hair from the dog that bites you will ease the pain of the bite. In hangover terms, the belief translates into the idea that having another drink counteracts symptoms caused by alcohol withdrawal and gets rid of the hangover. If it does have a beneficial effect on any of the other symptoms, it is only by decreasing your awareness of them. All another drink does is delay the inevitable. The hangover will return and will probably be even worse.

▶ Drinking a pint of water before you go to bed obviously helps prevent dehydration, but can also mean you getting up all through the night to go to the loo.

▶ Painkillers, such as aspirin, ibuprofen and paracetamol, can help to relieve the headache but do little else. Aspirin and ibuprofen can also inflame the lining of the stomach, so, if you are feeling a bit tender

Avoiding a hangover

★ Do not drink!
★ Avoid dark-coloured drinks.
★ Drink water throughout the evening.
★ Don't drink on an empty stomach.
★ Know your limits and stay within them.

If all this fails, and it often does, next morning do the following:

★ Avoid coffee – it just worsens the dehydration.
★ Take two paracetamol for the headache.
★ Take an antacid for a tender stomach.
★ Drink copious amounts of flat (not fizzy) soft drinks.
★ If you feel like eating, stick to starchy carbohydrates such as toast.
★ Stay in bed until the alcohol is out of your system.

in the morning, it is better to avoid these painkillers altogether.

▶ Vitamin C is included in some over-the-counter remedies, but there is little, if any, scientific evidence to prove it helps.

▶ Prairie Oyster – basically a spiced raw egg quaffed in one. I can think of no earthly reason why hangover 'cures' such as this one should work, although there may be some strange logic in the fact that by voluntarily forcing yourself to drink something so disgusting you might feel better – a variation of the no-pain-no-gain theory. I have never been that desperate, myself!

Sensible drinking: the current recommendations

The uncertainty surrounding precisely how much we can safely drink is reflected in the way that the guidelines have changed over the last few decades.

In 1979, the safe limits for both men and women were fifty-six units per week. These were lowered to fifty for men and thirty-five for women in 1986. Just a year later, doctors had another look and a working party of the Royal Colleges of General Practitioners, Psychiatrists and Physicians lowered the limits again. This time they defined safe limits as up to twenty-one units a week for men and up to fourteen units a week for women.

In the light of increasing evidence that moderate alcohol consumption (two to four units a day) may actually be beneficial in protecting us from heart disease, the limits were again reviewed in 1994 by the Royal Colleges of General Practitioners. However when the group reported back, it decided that there were insufficient grounds for raising drinking levels and reaffirmed the earlier sensible limits. Chairman of the working party, Professor Michael Marmot, said 'Giving everyone the green light to drink more would mean increasing risk of illness and death from causes other than coronary heart disease, and would significantly increase the risk of physical, mental and social damage from alcohol abuse as a whole.'

Despite this stance the Department of Health controversially opted to raise the limits to twenty-one units a week for women and twenty-eight units a week for men the following year and these are the

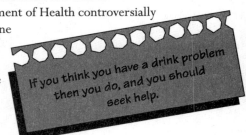

If you think you have a drink problem then you do, and you should seek help.

current recommendations. They come with the provision that 'at these levels most individuals are unlikely to come to any harm, provided the total amount is not drunk in one or two bouts and that there are occasional drink-free days'.

The Department of Health currently recommends no more than twenty-eight units of alcohol a week for men and twenty-one units a week for women.

If men are actually drinking between twenty-eight and forty units per week and women between twenty-one and thirty-five units, there is an increasing risk to their health. Above these limits they are almost certainly damaging their health and increasing their risk of becoming dependent on alcohol. The DoH's move to raise limits was virtually unaminously condemned by doctors.

Part of the problem is that the relationship between alcohol and disease or death is a very complex one, and we have to balance the recently discussed benefits against the hazard of people feeling encouraged to drink more. For example, the chances of a man, in his early twenties, dying of coronary heart disease is very rare, so telling him he can drink more is not likely to benefit him. In fact, the opposite is more likely to be true. His main cause of death, then, is likely to be from an accident or violence. Both these incidents are often alcohol related, and the more a young man drinks the more likely they are to happen. Similarly, when you consider all types of death in women, those who drink under one to two units a day are less likely to die than those who drink more.

However, as we get older, for example, men in their forties and women in their fifties, the risk of heart disease and stroke also goes up, so that the risk of encouraging light to moderate drinking begins to outweigh other risks, particularly for members of these groups who are at high risk of coronary heart disease, that is, if they smoke or have high blood pressure, etc. A recent study among British male doctors confirms that there is a net health benefit among light to moderate drinkers, including those who were drinking slightly above the twenty-one units a week in their seventies and eighties.

To sum up, whatever we read about the favourable benefits of alcohol, we need to bear in mind that there is no evidence of any health benefits from alcohol in anyone under forty. The other drawback of raising the limits is that already more than one in four men and one in ten women drink more than they should. There is a danger that raising the limits and stressing the health benefits of alcohol may just increase the number of people who exceeded the limits.

Alcohol and heart disease

Studies suggest that drinking moderate amounts of alcohol (two to four units a day) can protect against heart disease. Please note, however, that any less or more than this, is associated with an increased risk.

The protection is thought to be due to the effect that alcohol has on the types of cholesterol in the blood. Moderate amounts, as outlined above, increase the amount of good HDL cholesterol (see Cholesterol, Chapter One) which, in turn, reduces the likelihood of fat being deposited in the artery walls, leading to narrowing of the arteries and poor blood flow.

I have already mentioned the French Paradox (see page 159) and this apparent protection has been highlighted in work by a leading French

HAZARDS OF DRINKING

It is all very well to debate the possible advantages of moderate alcohol consumption, but there is absolutely no doubt about the disadvantages of drinking too much.

A UK Government-commissioned survey found that more than one in twenty men and one in one hundred women drink more than fifty units of alcohol a week. This means that as many as five million people in this country are likely to have an alcohol-related problem.

No part of the body is immune from the effects of heavy drinking. But the damage is not just physical, it can have profound emotional, social and psychological implications as well.

Physical consequences
★ Liver: hepatitis and cirrhosis.
★ Brain: memory loss, hallucinations, fits, confusion and loss of intellectual capability. ▷

◁ ★ Heart: damaged heart muscle and heart failure.
★ Stomach: heartburn, gastritis, ulcers and bleeding.
★ Pancreas: inflammation.
★ Cancer: mouth, throat and oesophagus.
★ Addiction: delirium tremens (DTs) and convulsions (fits) on withdrawal.
★ Malnutrition – heavy drinkers often neglect eating.
★ Infertility.

Social consequences
★ Problems at home.
★ Problems at work.
★ Problems with the law, for example drink-driving.
★ Violence.
★ Increased chance of accidents.

Psychological consequences
★ Effect on mood: euphoria, aggression (short term). Anxiety, panic attacks and depression (long term).
★ Effect on intellect: poor judgement, poor memory, and loss of protective inhibitions leading to unreasonable, unsafe and dangerous conduct.
★ Psychiatric effects: increased risk of suicide, paranoia, morbid jealousy, sexual problems and hallucinations.
★ Dependence: craving and loss of control.

researcher, Dr Serge Renaud. He has shown that drinking red wine can reduce the risk of heart disease by at least forty per cent. Indeed, he blames the high rate of heart disease in the UK on our comparatively low wine consumption.

When Dr Renaud appeared on American television in 1991 espousing his theory, sales of Pinot Noir and Zinfandel rose by thirty-nine per cent, Cabernet Sauvigon by

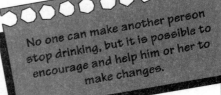

No one can make another person stop drinking, but it is possible to encourage and help him or her to make changes.

forty-three per cent and Merlot by eighty-three per cent. No wonder his recent trip to Britain was sponsored by the Bordeaux Wine Bureau. Call me a cynic if you like. However, it does appear that moderate alcohol consumption protects the heart but, to be perfectly honest, the medical evidence that red wine offers added benefit is not convincing.

The relationship between alcohol and disease or death is a very complex one.

Who is at risk?

It has long been recognised that heavy drinking tends to run in families. Recent work has suggested that this is partly due to an inherited tendency, and conditioning, over which we appear to have little control, and to environmental factors. In other words the son of a heavy drinker is more likely to be a heavy drinker himself because he has been bought up in a house where alcohol is an accepted part of life.

One in thirty of the general population can be classified as a problem drinker, but this figure rises to as many as one in four of the close relatives of problem drinkers.

Men are three times more likely to suffer alcohol related problems than women, but it now appears that women are starting to catch up.

Single people tend to be heavier drinkers than married people, and professional people drink more than unskilled manual workers (see Alcohol endangered professions, below). Predictably publicans top the league table – and doctors are not far behind.

Geographically, men in the north and north-west of Britain drink the most, and those in East Anglia the least.

Alcohol endangered professions

The charity, Alcohol Concern, has compiled the following list of what it calls dead-end jobs – those jobs with the highest death rates from alcohol related problems: publicans and bar staff, doctors, seafarers, lawyers, literary and artistic occupations, armed forces, fishing and related workers, caterers, dockers and goods' porter, cooks and kitchen porters.

Women show a slightly different pattern from the above list. Although female publicans and bar staff again appear to drink the most, they are followed by women in literary and artistic occupations and hairdressers.

Also, while the mortality rates provide one indicator of levels of drinking, they do not tell the whole story. For example, they do not reflect the recent changes in alcohol intake among today's generation of so-called yuppies. Study of the data from Alcohol Concern's General Households Survey on drinking levels revealed that in the professional groups – including the legal profession, accountants and senior executives – heavy drinking in the younger age group is well above the population average, with more than sixteen per cent of young men, and over seven per cent of young women, drinking more than the safe limit.

When is someone a problem drinker?

The moment a doctor suggests to a patient that their health is suffering as a result of drinking, most become very defensive and immediately deny that they are an alcoholic.

Many doctors no longer use the term alcoholic because it carries with it

WHAT ARE THE WARNING SIGNS OF ALCOHOL DEPENDENCE?

★ Alcohol starts to take priority over everything else, including family, partners, friends, work, social life and eating.

★ Drinking becomes secretive and the general behaviour of the drinker becomes dishonest and deceitful.

★ Memory lapses, particularly relating to the previous night's activities, become common.

★ Increased tolerance to drink creates the need to drink more to have the same effect.

★ Withdrawal symptoms caused by a drop in blood alcohol levels are accompanied by symptoms such as morning shakes, agitation, nausea and sweating. More alcohol is believed to be the only 'cure'. The person increasingly needs alcohol to function normally and will suffer craving if they try to abstain.

the mistaken idea that the condition is irreversible and untreatable. Indeed, just labelling someone an alcoholic can be enough to prevent the person seeking help for a drink problem.

In my experience, dividing drinkers into those who drink moderate amounts and those who are 'alcoholics' encourages many people to think that they can drink what they like, and provided they are not classified as an alcoholic they will not have any problems. Nothing could be farther from the truth. Anyone who has a physical, emotional, social or psychological problem as a result of drinking alcohol has a drink problem. A person does not need to be addicted to, or dependent on, alcohol to have a drink problem, but those who are, usually suffer serious problems as a result. It is this latter group that are commonly referred to as alcoholics.

WHAT TO DO WHEN SOMEONE IS DRINKING TOO MUCH

★ Talk to the person when they are sober and you are reasonably calm. Avoid getting into arguments. Be consistent in what you say and do. Never say one thing and do another. Listen to them when they explain why they think drink is helping them.

★ Tell them about the problems their drinking is causing to others.

★ Make clear what behaviour you will not accept and what action you will take if it continues. Never make idle threats.

★ Tell other members of the family what you are doing.

★ Help the person who is drinking to be realistic and face up to the problems.

★ Don't make it easy for them to drink and never buy alcohol for them.

★ Help the person to see the effects that heavy drinking is having both on themselves and others.

★ Don't hide the effects of the problem from the drinker or from other people.

★ Be aware that changing drinking habits can be a long process and that there are bound to be many problems, including relapses, along the way.

Acknowledging a drink problem

More often than not alcohol dependent drinkers avoid talking about their problem and, when questioned, will deny that they have one. This means they rarely come to the attention of their doctors unless problems in their life force them to do so. Matters may also come to a head when the partner, often the wife, visits the surgery to get help.

No one can make another person stop drinking, but it is possible to encourage and help him or her to make changes (see What to do when someone is drinking too much, opposite). The first step is to get the person to acknowledge the problem. The second stage is for the individual to start controlling the drink or to undergo complete abstinence.

Alcoholics, by definition, cannot control their drinking and total abstinence is often the only option. Stopping drinking can lead to quite marked side-effects and needs to be done under medical supervision. Once the person has stopped drinking, support and follow-up care are vital. Their families also need support and follow-up care and should not be neglected.

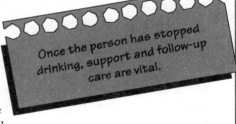

Once the person has stopped drinking, support and follow-up care are vital.

What to do if you are the problem drinker

If you think you have a drink problem then you do, and you should seek help. There are a number of options available.

The first is to tell your partner, if you have one. Almost certainly he or she will be fully aware of what is going on and will be greatly relieved that you are coming to terms with the problem.

The next step is to see your GP who will assess what, if any, physical damage you have done to yourself, and offer counselling and advice. If you do not want to speak to your GP about this problem but would like to find out what help is available, contact Drinkline, a national alcohol helpline, that offers confidential information and advice.

For more detailed counselling and support, go direct to a self-help group, such as Alcoholics Anonymous (AA). Do not be put off by the use of the term alcoholic. AA will help anyone who feels they have a drink problem, no matter how large or small.

Most areas in the country have a drop-in community alcohol unit. Your GP will have details of your nearest unit, but you can contact it direct or just turn up in person. The telephone number and address should be under Alcohol in the telephone directory.

✉ Useful addresses

▶ Accept Services UK, 724 Fulham Road, London SW6 5SE. Telephone: 0171 371 7477. Offer advice and information and run group therapy sessions. Send a sae for leaflets.

▶ AL-Anon Family Groups, 61 Great Dover Street, London SE1 4YF. Telephone: 0171 403 0888. This is a self-help group for the family and close associates of problem drinkers.

▶ Alateen, Address as AL-Anon above. Similar to AL-Anon, but for teenage children of problem drinkers.

▶ Adult Children of Alcoholics, PO Box 1576, London SW3 1AZ. Telephone: 0171 229 4587.

▶ Alcoholics Anonymous (AA), PO Box 1, Stonebow House, Stonebow, York YO1 2NJ. Telephone: 01904 644026/7/8/9. AA is a fellowship of nearly 200 groups in the UK. The aim is for the person to give up alcohol entirely. Members meet to share experiences and help each other. Local groups are usually listed in the telephone directory.

▶ Alcohol Concern, Waterbridge House, 32–6 Loman Street, London SE1 0EE. Telephone: 0171 928 7377. Alcohol Concern is a national charity dealing with drink problems.

▶ Drinkline: The National Alcohol Helpline. Open evenings from 6 p.m. to 11 p.m. Telephone: 0171 332 0202. They give confidential information and advice, and can put individuals in touch with local advice centres.

FURTHER READING

FOOD

Diet Breaking (having it all without having to diet) – Mary Evans Young (Hodder & Stoughton, 1995)

The Good Diet – Jane Dunkeld (Robinson Publishing Ltd, 1995)

You Don't Have to Diet: dieting is not the solution...it's the problem – Dr Tom Sanders and Peter Bazalgette (Bantam Press,)

The Complete BBC Diet – Dr Barry Lynch (BBC Books/Penguin, 1994)

Peter Cox's Guide to Vegetarian Living – Peter Cox (Bloomsbury, 1995)

Reader's Digest Foods that Harm, Foods that Heal – The Reader's Digest Association Ltd (1996)

SKIN

Skin Problems: a self-help guide – Hasnain Walji and Dr Andrea Kingston (Hodder & Stoughton, 1994)

STRESS

Laughter, the best medicine: the healing power of happiness, humour and laughter – Robert Holden (Thorsons, 1993)

Stress Busters: over 100 successful strategies for stress survival – Robert Holden (Thorsons, 1992)

SMOKING

The Smoker's Health Plan – Dr James Scala (Thorsons, 1993)

ALCOHOL

The Recovery Book: a life-saving guide for recovering alcoholics, addicts and their families – Al J. Mooney, Arlene Eisenberg and Howard Bisenberg (Robinson Publishing Ltd, 1995)

SLEEP

The New Natural Family Doctor: the authoritative self-help guide to health and natural medicine – General Editor: Dr Andrew Stanway (Gaia Books Ltd, 1996)

The Good Sleep Guide – Michael van Straten (Kyle Cathie Ltd, 1996)

INDEX

Index